A PLAGUE ON
ALL OUR HOUSES

BRUCE J. HILLMAN, MD

A Plague
on All Our
Houses

MEDICAL INTRIGUE, HOLLYWOOD,

AND THE DISCOVERY OF AIDS

ForeEdge

ForeEdge

An imprint of University Press of New England

www.upne.com

© 2017 Bruce J. Hillman

All rights reserved

Manufactured in the United States of America

Designed by Mindy Basinger Hill

Typeset in Fresco Plus Pro

For permission to reproduce any of the material in this book,
contact Permissions, University Press of New England, One Court Street,
Suite 250, Lebanon NH 03766; or visit www.upne.com

Library of Congress Cataloging-in-Publication Data

Names: Hillman, Bruce J., author.

Title: A plague on all our houses: medical intrigue, Hollywood,
and the discovery of AIDS / Bruce J. Hillman.

Description: Lebanon NH: ForeEdge, [2016] |
Includes bibliographical references and index.

Identifiers: LCCN 2016006933 (print) | LCCN 2016008228 (ebook) |
ISBN 9781611688757 (cloth) | ISBN 9781611689969 (epub, mobi & pdf)

Subjects: | MESH: Gottlieb, Michael S. | Faculty, Medical | HIV Infections—history
| Social Conditions—history | Education, Medical, Graduate—history | Schools,
Medical—history | Politics | History, 20th Century | Biography

Classification: LCC RA643.8 (print) | LCC RA643.8 (ebook) |
NLM WZ 100 | DDC 614.5/99392—dc23
LC record available at http://lccn.loc.gov/2016006933

5   4   3   2   1

For those who died from bigotry, ignorance, and neglect

For those who survived because of advocacy and scientific investigation

and

For those dedicated to improving prevention and finding a cure

CONTENTS

On July 5, 1981, the world was made aware of a seemingly small but ultimately very important bit of new knowledge. Barely noticed at first, Dr. Michael Gottlieb's communication in *Morbidity and Mortality Weekly Report* (MMWR) about five gay men with a mysterious and deadly new disease announced the beginning of the worldwide AIDS epidemic.

Gottlieb's patients were not the very first cases of AIDS. Other physicians had been seeing patients with AIDS for a decade or more.[1] His contribution was that he made the intellectual leap. He was the first to recognize that what he and others were seeing was a new and dangerous disease. Gottlieb was the first to publish the constellation of physical and laboratory findings of AIDS, expanding on our understanding later in 1981 with an article in the *New England Journal of Medicine* (NEJM) that is now recognized as a classic. In 2011 the NEJM chose Gottlieb's article as one of just a handful of "Historical Journal Articles Cited" over the two-hundred-year history of the journal.[2]

More than thirty-five years after that publication, the worldwide epidemic continues unabated. AIDS afflicts gay and straight, men and women, children and adults. Health-care providers in the United States report fifty thousand new cases of HIV infection annually. While years of research have led to drug therapies that extend patients' lives, scientists have yet to devise either a curative treatment or a preventative vaccine. For less developed societies, the situation is much worse. Modern pharmaceuticals are not reliably available, and AIDS remains a leading cause of illness and death in the Third World.

A great deal has been written about AIDS. Library shelves sag under the weight of scientific treatises, memoirs, and histories. So why would I or anyone else write another book about AIDS? What distinguishes *A Plague on All Our Houses* is its perspective. Rather than trying to write another comprehensive history, I have focused the narrative on AIDS discoverer Dr. Michael Gottlieb and on those whose actions influenced his thoughts and experiences. Guided primarily by my interviews with Dr. Gottlieb and many others who played important roles during the early years of the epidemic, the book diverges from the journalistic approach of such classics as Randy Shilts's *And the Band Played On* to explore a much more personal story. From Gottlieb's first scientific publication on the new immunologic malady in 1981 to 1988, when a Job-like convergence of personal and professional challenges forced him into a self-defining Hobson's choice, readers confront the opportunities and challenges Gottlieb encountered as he and his contemporaries experienced them.

Foremost among my several objectives in writing this book was to tell an interesting and instructive story, to provide a nonfiction account of an important era that would read like a fiction page-turner. At its heart, *Plague* is a story about an individual's conflict with a powerful system. In 1981 Gottlieb was a newly minted, untenured assistant professor whose discovery launched his career on a meteoric course and set prodigious expectations.

In setting out to fulfill his promise, Gottlieb was motivated by a sincere desire to improve upon the dismal lot of those afflicted with the new disease. However, this is not to say that altruism was his only motivation. Gottlieb was an ambitious young physician intent on building a successful, indeed a noteworthy, academic career. Well-intentioned in pursuing the cause of HIV/AIDS patients, but unprepared for the intense academic infighting that followed his discovery, Gottlieb made decisions that progressively put him at odds with his immediate bosses and the institutional administration and isolated him from his colleagues.

Another of my objectives in writing *Plague* was to invite readers to peek into the scantly explored world of university physicians, where I have persisted and thrived for nearly forty years. The public image of an academic physician, if one exists at all, is of a tolerant, middle-aged-going-on-elderly professor teaching admiring acolytes in a plummy, vaguely British-sounding accent. Nothing could be further from reality. Academic medicine is highly competitive. There are winners and losers, and the survivors typically show little sympathy for those who fall by the wayside. Following Dr. Gottlieb's path through the labyrinthine cultural mores of academe provides a glimpse of how academic medicine works and to what ends.

I also wanted to place the discovery and early years of AIDS in the context of the times. To paint the political and cultural backdrop of the 1980s without interrupting the main story line, I have inserted at intervals throughout the book short chapters featuring a patient whom I have named Brad Hartley. Hartley is a well-educated and thoughtful gay man who, when he first appears in the book, worriedly seeks Gottlieb's professional advice about how his promiscuous lifestyle might affect his risk of contracting AIDS. Through Hartley's interactions with Gottlieb and his evolving perspective on key events over the same time frame as the main narrative, I hope readers will gain an appreciation of how politics, religion, and the arts impacted public attitudes toward AIDS. As this is a work of nonfiction, all of the events presented in the Hartley chapters did occur. However, to preserve the anonymity of my sources and save them the risk of possible embarrassment, "Brad Hartley" is an amalgam, sometimes expressing the thoughts and experiences of one individual and at other times those of another.

In writing *A Plague on All Our Houses,* I pieced together bits of information from various sources to present the most accurate history I could. These included previously published books and magazine articles, a host of Web pages, and documents shared with me by their owners. However, the most critical sources, without which this book would not have been possible, are my interviews with the people who lived this history. Nearly all of the men and women who figure importantly in this story are still alive. Almost everyone I contacted generously agreed to speak with me for one or more interviews and to respond to follow-up questions as needed.

I honestly believe that everyone with whom I spoke told me about the events detailed in this book according to his or her best recollections. However, in some important instances there were key differences in what two or more people remembered. When there was substantive disagreement on pivotal issues, I did the best I could to identify additional individuals who might have firsthand knowledge of events, to inform what properly should be incorporated into the book. When this was not possible, I tried to be as evenhanded as possible in presenting the disparate impressions of those involved.

Finally, our society's experience in dealing with the early years of the AIDS epidemic has much to teach us about how to approach new outbreaks of infectious diseases as they pop up around the globe. From our relatively safe perch in the United States, it is easy to forget that the majority of the world's population still periodically suffers flare-ups of infectious diseases that kill thousands in a single stroke. To ignore the disparity would be irresponsible. Moreover, the flattening of our planet by air travel and telecommunications; the insanity of parents refusing to inoculate their children against once common infectious diseases; and factors encouraging the persistence of poverty, unsanitary conditions, and malnutrition anywhere in the world portend the very real possibility that diseases we once thought conquered will once again find fertile ground here in the United States and wreak havoc on our immunologically naive population. The 2014–2015 epidemic of Ebola in West Africa teaches us that no one is truly safe from the ravages of epidemic infectious disease. The current status of AIDS worldwide and how our experience with the AIDS epidemic should inform policy to better prepare us for future epidemics are further detailed in the epilogue.

The story of the discovery of AIDS and the events that followed is an instructive and cautionary tale about the soured fruits of pride, envy among colleagues, and dashed hopes redeemed by self-examination and reinvention. I am indebted to Dr. Michael Gottlieb, who attended medical school with me at the University of Rochester. Dr. Gottlieb spent countless hours in conversation with me, sometimes straining to retrieve recollections of events he had not thought about for many years. Without his cooperation, this book would not have been possible.

I also thank the many others who provided their invaluable insights. (Please see my acknowledgments at the end of this book.) Their reminiscences helped round out, give credence to, or in some cases contradict the recollections of Dr. Gottlieb and the others I interviewed. In taking everyone's memories of that time into account, I made what I believe were the best possible efforts to honestly and evenhandedly portray events as they occurred. In the end, all decisions concerning what material appears in *A Plague on All Our Houses* and what ended up on the cutting table are my own. I am solely responsible for the contents of this book. I apologize in advance for any errors of fact or interpretation.

DRAMATIS PERSONAE

Sheldon Andelson—Philanthropist and member of the California Board
of Regents, whom Dr. Gottlieb viewed as being sympathetic to his
goals.

Françoise Barré-Sinoussi—Researcher at the Pasteur Institute in Paris
who, along with senior researcher Luc Montagnier, discovered
the virus responsible for causing AIDS.

David Barry, MD—Senior researcher and head of virology research at
Burroughs Wellcome pharmaceutical company, who was responsible for bringing AZT to FDA approval.

Samuel Broder, MD—Senior researcher at the National Cancer Institute
and the principal researcher in the pivotal trial leading to the
FDA's approval of AZT.

Willie Brown—California legislator and speaker of the State Assembly,
who helped direct state funding for AIDS research to the University of California San Francisco and UCLA.

Harold Burger, MD, PhD—Virologist at Stanford who had been among
those working on elucidating the cause of AIDS.

Letantia Bussell, MD—Beverly Hills dermatologist who referred Rock
Hudson to Dr. Gottlieb to confirm her diagnosis of HIV/AIDS and
provide AIDS-related care.

Jonathan Canno—Member of Dr. Krim's AMF board of directors and
long-term amfAR board member, instrumental in consummating
the AMF merger with Dr. Gottlieb's NARF.

Jean-Claude Chermann—AIDS researcher working in the laboratory of
Dr. Luc Montagnier.

Marcus Conant, MD—San Francisco AIDS researcher who helped steer
California legislature-mandated funding for AIDS research to Dr.
Gottlieb.

John Crewdson—*Chicago Tribune* investigative reporter, who wrote a nearly book-length article for the newspaper exposing ethical concerns about the work of Dr. Robert Gallo.

Bruce Decker—Well-known AIDS advocate and friend of Dr. Gottlieb, who served with him on the California AIDS Advisory Committee and who first told him about Dr. Krim's interest in merging her foundation with his.

Joseph Elia, MD—Associate editor of the *New England Journal of Medicine*, who fielded Dr. Gottlieb's call inquiring about the journal's interest in his discovery of a new immune disease.

John Fahey, MD, PhD—Renowned immunologist and colleague of Drs. Gottlieb and Saxon in the UCLA Division of Clinical Immunology and Allergy.

Peng Fan, MD—Interim head of rheumatology at the Wadsworth Veterans Administration Medical Center, who brokered Dr. Joel Weisman's referral of two AIDS patients to Dr. Gottlieb.

Anthony Fauci, MD—Infectious disease specialist and director of the National Institute of Allergy and Infectious Disease.

Margaret Fischl, MD—AIDS researcher and head of the AIDS Clinical Research Unit at the University of Miami.

Kevin Robert Frost—CEO of amfAR.

Robert Gallo, MD—Leading National Institutes of Health researcher, who described the first retrovirus. His lab competed with the Pasteur Institute researchers who ultimately were credited with discovering the virus that causes AIDS.

David Geffen—Los Angeles entertainment impresario who favored merging Gottlieb's NARF and Krim's AMF, and who was part of the conversations leading up to the merger.

David Golde, MD—Head of the Division of Oncology in the UCLA Department of Medicine.

Michael Gottlieb, MD—Assistant professor of medicine in the Division of Clinical Immunology and Allergy at UCLA, who in 1981 discovered a new viral disease now called AIDS.

Paul Gottlieb—Dr. Gottlieb's older brother.

Steven Gottlieb—Dr. Gottlieb's younger brother.

Jerome Groopman, MD—UCLA and later Harvard oncologist, who was
   Gottlieb's original partner in the UCLA AIDS Center, specializing
   in the cancers associated with AIDS.

Brad Hartley—A composite of several AIDS patients with experiences
   pertinent to the time period covered by the book.

Rock Hudson—Film star and patient of Dr. Gottlieb. He was the first celebrity to admit to having AIDS and died from the condition.

Ross Hunter—Movie director and friend of Rock Hudson.

Rex Kenemer, MD—Rock Hudson's primary physician.

Arnold Klein, MD—Los Angeles dermatologist who was active in the negotiations merging Dr. Gottlieb's NARF and Dr. Krim's AMF.

C. Everett Koop, MD—Surgeon General of the United States.

Larry Kramer—Author, artist, playwright, and gay rights advocate inti-
   mately involved in the origination of ACT UP; author of the play
   The Normal Heart.

Arthur Krim—Film mogul who served on the boards of AMF and then
   amfAR, and husband of Mathilde Krim.

Mathilde Krim, PhD—New York socialite and AIDS advocate who, with
   Elizabeth Taylor and Dr. Gottlieb, cofounded amfAR. For many
   years she served as the chair of amfAR's board of directors.

Lyndon LaRouche—California politician who initiated the Proposition
   64 movement.

Jay Levy, MD—University of California San Francisco AIDS researcher.

Mark Miller—Rock Hudson's personal assistant.

Bill Misenhimer—Former Xerox financial executive who became the executive director of AIDS Project Los Angeles and then of amfAR.

Ronald Mitsuyasu, MD—Assistant professor in the UCLA Department
   of Medicine's Division of Oncology, who assumed responsibility
   for patients with the cancer-related manifestations of AIDS at the
   UCLA AIDS Center following Dr. Jerome Groopman's departure.

Luc Montagnier, MD, PhD—Senior researcher at the Pasteur Institute,
   who along with his colleague, Dr. Barré-Sinoussi, is credited with
   the discovery of the virus that causes AIDS.

Harry Nelson—Science and health reporter for the *Los Angeles Times*.

Dale Olson—Rock Hudson's publicist.

Kathy Petersilie—Laboratory assistant to Dr. Gottlieb.

John Pontarelli—Director of public relations for UCLA Medical Center.

Arnold Relman, MD—Editor of the *New England Journal of Medicine*, who advised Dr. Gottlieb on how he should manage his new discovery.

Pierre Salinger—ABC chief foreign correspondent. He arranged for Rock Hudson's flight home from Paris following his diagnosis of AIDS.

Chen Sam—Elizabeth Taylor's publicist.

Greg Sarna, MD—UCLA lymphoma specialist whom Dr. Gottlieb consulted to verify Rock Hudson's diagnosis and suggest a course of action.

Andrew Saxon, MD, PhD—Head of the Division of Clinical Immunology and Allergy at UCLA and Dr. Gottlieb's immediate superior.

Howard Schanker, MD—Clinical fellow working under Dr. Gottlieb in the Division of Clinical Immunology and Allergy at UCLA.

Robert Schroff, PhD—Postdoctoral student conducting research under the guidance of Dr. John Fahey in the Division of Clinical Immunology and Allergy at UCLA. He conducted the tests that identified the immunologic abnormality characteristically seen in patients with AIDS.

Steve Schulte—Director of the Los Angeles Gay and Lesbian Service Center.

Wayne Shandara, MD—Centers for Disease Control epidemic intelligence service officer assigned to the LA County Health Department. He investigated Dr. Gottlieb's concern about the outbreak of a new immunologic disease and worked with him on writing the first article to be published about AIDS.

Martin Shapiro, MD—Head of the Division of General Medicine, a division of the Department of Medicine at UCLA.

Wally Sheft—Rock Hudson's business manager and accountant, who served as intermediary for Hudson's donation to Dr. Gottlieb to use in starting a foundation to enhance AIDS research.

Kenneth Shine, MD—Chairman of the UCLA Department of Medicine, responsible for oversight of all the divisions of the department and the immediate superior of Dr. Andrew Saxon.

Frederick Siegal, MD—New York physician who, along with Henry Masur, reported cases of what is now known as AIDS in the same issue of the *New England Journal of Medicine* as Dr. Gottlieb.

Ake Spross—A reporter for the Swedish daily newspaper *Upsala Nya Tidning* and e-mail correspondent of Dr. Gottlieb.

Elizabeth Taylor—Noted film actress and one of the founders of amfAR, along with Drs. Michael Gottlieb and Mathilde Krim. She also founded the Elizabeth Taylor AIDS Foundation.

Jay Theodore—Administrative assistant to Dr. Gottlieb.

Brad Volkmer—UCLA Medical Center administrator to whom Dr. Gottlieb appealed for office and research space.

Roger Wall—Elizabeth Taylor's personal assistant.

Henry Waxman—California congressman who was the leading spokesman for federal funding of AIDS research during the 1980s.

Herbert Weiner, MD—Noted UCLA professor of psychiatry and therapist to Dr. Gottlieb.

Joel Weisman, DO—Openly gay private practice physician in the San Fernando Valley, whose medical practice included a significant number of gay patients with HIV/AIDS. He also served on the amfAR board of directors.

Cindy Wheelhouse—Michael Gottlieb's first wife; now Cindy Sapp.

Barbara Weiser, MD, BH—Virologist at Stanford who was among those working on elucidating the cause of AIDS.

Robert Wolf, MD—Medical intern in the UCLA Department of Medicine who admitted to the hospital and cared for the first case of AIDS and referred the patient to Dr. Gottlieb.

Peter Wolfe, MD—Colleague of Dr. Gottlieb in the Division of Clinical Immunology and Allergy at UCLA.

Harald zur Hausen, MD, PhD—Discoverer of the human papilloma virus and 2008 Nobel laureate along with Drs. Montagenier and Barré-Sinnousi.

GLOSSARY OF INSTITUTES,
DEPARTMENTS, AND FOUNDATIONS

AIDS Center—Entity under which Dr. Gottlieb initially provided clinical care for patients with HIV/AIDS in UCLA's outpatient clinical facilities.

AIDS Clinical Research Center—Entity Dr. Gottlieb founded and directed at UCLA, based on California legislative funding of AIDS research, beginning in 1983.

AIDS Medical Foundation (AMF)—Entity founded by Dr. Mathilde Krim to provide grants for AIDS research and perform advocacy work on behalf of AIDS. It merged with Dr. Gottlieb's National AIDS Research Foundation (NARF) to form amfAR.

AIDS Project Los Angeles—Small, poorly funded local organization providing support services to the Los Angeles gay community, which under its executive director, Bill Misenhimer, grew to prominence through its annual Commitment to Life gala.

AIDS Treatment Evaluation Unit—Reorganization proposed by Dr. Gottlieb to enable UCLA to fulfill its responsibilities under his successful proposal for NIAID funding.

American Foundation for AIDS Research (amfAR)—Entity formed by the merger of Dr. Gottlieb's National AIDS Research Foundation and Dr. Krim's AIDS Medical Foundation.

Centers for Disease Control (CDC)—Federal agency responsible for, among other things, the investigation of outbreaks of disease within the United States.

Department of Medicine—Department of the UCLA School of Medicine responsible for the provision of care; teaching of medical students, residents, fellows, and practicing physicians; and conducting biomedical research with respect to internal medicine. Its chair oversaw numerous divisions, including the Division of Clinical Immunology and Allergy.

Division of Clinical Immunology and Allergy (CIA)—Division of the
UCLA Department of Medicine, headed by Dr. Andrew Saxon.

Elizabeth Taylor AIDS Foundation (ETAF)—Entity established in 1991 to
provide small grants to organizations serving the needs of AIDS
patients.

Global AIDS Interfaith Alliance (GAIA)—Organization that provides AIDS
and medical support services to rural African villages.

Morbidity and Mortality Weekly Report (MMWR)—Centers for Disease
Control publication in which Dr. Gottlieb first published case reports of patients with AIDS.

National AIDS Research Foundation (NARF)—Entity founded by Dr.
Gottlieb to award grants to AIDS researchers. Before it became
active, NARF merged with Dr. Krim's AMF to form amfAR.

National Cancer Institute (NCI)—Institute of the National Institutes of
Health responsible for research and other activities related to cancer.

National Institute of Allergy and Infectious Diseases (NIAID)—Institute
of the National Institutes of Health responsible for research and
other activities related to allergies and infectious diseases.

National Institutes of Health (NIH)—Twenty-seven government institutes and centers responsible for conducting research, establishing consensus on best medical practices, and communicating
with health-care providers and the public concerning related diseases and technologies.

National Institutes of Health Clinical Research Center—Medical care
facility on the NIH campus providing inpatient and outpatient clinical and support services for patients participating in
NIH-sponsored clinical trials.

New England Journal of Medicine (NEJM)—Prestigious medical publication in which Dr. Gottlieb published his series of reports on AIDS
cases and its primary cellular abnormality of low counts of CD4
T-lymphocytes.

Wadsworth Veterans Administration Hospital—UCLA-affiliated teaching hospital at which Dr. Gottlieb had his office during the latter
part of his employment at UCLA.

A PLAGUE ON
ALL OUR HOUSES

One Sick Queen

Dr. Michael Gottlieb lifted his eyes from the patient's chart he was reviewing and waved his fellow, Howard Schanker, into his tiny basement office. He shoved aside a short stack of journals to clear a space for his younger colleague to sit, then listened as Schanker's Bronx-tinged voice detailed what he had learned about a patient he had discussed with a medical intern, Dr. Robert Wolf.[1] Their conversation set in motion a chain of events leading to Gottlieb's discovery of a new, previously undetected disease that in short order would engulf the entire world in a deadly epidemic that persists to the present day.

Wolf had admitted his patient to the hospital through the University of California Los Angeles emergency room. Baffled by the patient's constellation of findings, Wolf presented the case to the chair of UCLA's Department of Medicine, Dr. Kenneth Shine, during Shine's weekly clinical teaching rounds. Shine suggested that Wolf contact Dr. Gottlieb, a newly hired assistant professor who specialized in immunology.[2] The timing was perfect, as Gottlieb had recently asked Schanker to keep an eye out for new patients who might be suitable for his immunology teaching sessions with medical students and house staff.

Dr. Gottlieb was sufficiently intrigued by what Schanker told him that he immediately accompanied him to the patient's bedside so that he could personally assess the man's clinical findings. What Gottlieb saw was a thin, very ill-looking, thirty-year-old man, whose close-cut, bottle-blonde hair accentuated his haggard appearance.

The patient told Gottlieb that he had been in perfect health until roughly a month earlier, when he had rapidly become ill. He reported suffering from fever and reckoned that he had lost more than thirty pounds, at least in part because a sore throat made swallowing food excruciatingly painful. He was discomforted by skin ulcerations surrounding his anus.

Gottlieb ascertained that both the sore throat and the perianal ulcerations were caused by infections of the fungus *Candida albicans*, or
"thrush." *Candida* also was cultured from the patient's fingertips, although
only superficially, as the underlying abnormality was herpetic whitlow.[3]
Candida is ubiquitous in nature, but actual clinical infection is strictly
"opportunistic," meaning that illness only occurs in individuals who have
a deficient immune system, like some patients undergoing treatment for
cancer or taking drugs to prevent rejection of a transplanted organ. This
patient fit into neither category.

"The case smelled like an immune deficiency," said Gottlieb. "You don't
get a mouth full of *Candida* without being immune deficient."

There were other signs that the man's immune system was operating at
less than full capacity. Wolf had done skin testing for reactions to common
allergens that had failed to elicit any response. Blood tests had shown higher
than normal levels of certain types of antibodies circulating in his blood.
Clearly, Wolf's patient was confronting a serious challenge to his immunity.
However, contrary to what Gottlieb would have expected in a man fighting
off serious infections, his white blood cell count was well below normal.
Particularly depressed was the number of T-lymphocytes, a type of white
blood cell that helps the body eliminate dangerous invaders like bacteria and
fungi through a process known as "cell-mediated" or "cellular" immunity.

The patient improved with treatment for the fungal infection and was
discharged from the hospital, but returned one evening about a week later
with a hacking cough and difficulty catching his breath. Dr. Wolf happened
to be the intern who was next up to accept an admission. He resumed his
care of the patient and ordered a chest X-ray, which the radiologist interpreted as showing an interstitial pneumonia.[4] To Wolf, there were only
two possible causes for such a pattern: *Cytomegalovirus*, a viral infection for
which there was no treatment, and *Pneumocystis carinii*, an opportunistic
bacterial infection. In desperation, fearing that without treatment his patient would die, Wolf decided on his own to empirically initiate intravenous
Bactrim, a sulfa-class antibiotic known to be effective against *Pneumocystis*
pneumonia. Although this initially outraged Wolf's superiors as inappropriate without first obtaining proof of the responsible organism, the patient

rapidly improved. A subsequent lung biopsy confirmed that his pneumonia was, indeed, caused by the microorganism *Pneumocystis carinii*.[5]

Gottlieb and Schanker visited the man regularly during their morning rounds when they also saw their other patients to evaluate their progress, order tests, and make any necessary changes in their treatment. "Periodically, I'd hold immunology teaching rounds," Gottlieb said. "There would be ten or twelve of us—medical students, residents, and fellows—going room to room like a small army. One day, we all entered his room, and he was on the telephone with a friend, and he said to his friend, in jest, 'Hey, yes, Bruce, the doctors here tell me I am one sick queen!'[6] And we all chuckled because we were still very much in the dark about lifestyle issues and clueless when it came to self-deprecating gay humor." The moment of levity stirred Schanker's creativity. For some time thereafter, when Gottlieb and his fellow discussed the patient or encountered new cases with similar findings, Schanker insisted on calling the array of abnormalities "sick queen immune deficiency syndrome," or for brevity's sake, "SQUIDS." Dr. Wolf recalled that the unfortunate acronym began to spread among the house staff and soon appeared in patients' charts. The Department of Medicine finally put its foot down, circulating a memo that banned "SQUIDS" from further use.

When Gottlieb first heard about Wolf's patient in March 1981, the thirty-three-year-old physician was less than a year out of fellowship training and was newly employed as an assistant professor in the Division of Clinical Immunology and Allergy (CIA) at the UCLA School of Medicine. The division's personnel occupied a below-ground warren of windowless, cubby-hole offices and labs in one corner of the hospital, on what was known as A-Level. By what turned out to be an extraordinary stroke of serendipity, working in the lab across the hall from Gottlieb's office was Dr. Robert Schroff, a postdoctoral research fellow conducting investigations under the guidance of the eminent immunologist Dr. John Fahey. Schroff was testing a set of monoclonal antibodies[7] that attached to specific subtypes of T-lymphocytes, the very kind of white blood cell in which the patient was deficient. Gottlieb asked Schanker to have blood drawn for Schroff to conduct his analysis.

Since Gottlieb and Schanker were consultants, not the physicians primarily caring for the patient, protocol required that Schanker ask for the approval of the physician of record, Dr. Wolf. Wolf and his patient had bonded during the man's close brush with death. The patient put his complete trust in Wolf, who had grown up in the same St. Louis neighborhood and whom he believed had saved his life. Wolf agreed to collect the needed blood samples but exacted from Schanker a quid pro quo. Feeling that he had played a significant role in bringing the patient to Schanker's attention, Wolf asked that he be included as an author on any journal article reporting on his patient. Schanker agreed and returned to the lab with several tubes of blood.

Schroff's analysis revealed the principal immunologic abnormality caused by the condition now known as AIDS: a severe paucity of what were then called "helper T-cells" (now known as CD4 T-lymphocytes), which activate cellular immunity. In addition, the number of "suppressor T-cells" (CD8 T-lymphocytes), which help diminish the immune response, was very high. This peaked Gottlieb's interest.

"Now my bias had always been toward suppressor cells, because in the mid- to late-70s [when I was a fellow in immunology at Stanford University], suppressor cells were all the rage—that some diseases occurred because of an excess of T-cell suppression."[8] Thus, when Gottlieb looked at the data, his interest in diseases of immune suppression led him to think that the high level of suppressor cells was the cause of the disorder. His patient's inability to appropriately respond to opportunistic pathogens like *Candida* was compromised by the overload of suppressor T-cells. It wasn't until he had discussed the findings with senior immunologist John Fahey that he realized that he might be blindly focusing on suppressor cells when in fact it was the deficient helper T-cells that were truly at the root of the problem.

In short order, two additional patients with similar findings were referred to Gottlieb for consultation by Dr. Joel Weisman, who practiced in the San Fernando Valley, while a fourth patient was admitted to UCLA via the emergency room. Weisman was an openly gay osteopathic physician who had a largely gay practice in Sherman Oaks. Dr. Peng Fan, the interim head of rheumatology at the Wadsworth Veterans Administration Hospital—an affiliated teaching hospital of UCLA—was moonlighting at Riverside Hospital in the Valley to make a little extra money when he came across Weisman's patients. Fan convinced Weisman to drive into Los Angeles and discuss the cases with Gottlieb. Although initially wary of putting his gay patients in the hands of a straight physician, Weisman's concerns were assuaged when he learned that he and Gottlieb had grown up in the same part of New Jersey and had friends in common. Weisman ultimately agreed to transfer his patients to UCLA and place the two men under Gottlieb's care.

A single mysterious case of unexplained opportunistic infection was one thing, but four within such a short period of time was quite another. *What am I missing?* Gottlieb wondered. *Is the answer staring me in the face?* He considered the similarities among his patients. All of the men were in their thirties. They had initially presented with or soon developed rare, opportunistic infections. He had successfully treated the individual infections, at least for a while, yet his patients had uniformly deteriorated before his eyes. They all had shown the same depletion of the CD4 subtype of T-lymphocytes. And there was one more thing that the patients had in common: they were exclusively gay.

Deep in thought, Gottlieb halfheartedly riffled through the uneven stacks of journal articles and handwritten notes that all but obscured the surface of his desk. He rolled the chair bearing his six-foot frame backward until the soft brown curls covering his head touched the wall, then stretched his arms as far as they would go above his head to relieve the strained muscles in his back and neck. Wiping the oversized lenses of his long-outdated glasses, he thought to himself, *get back to basics.* He scanned the review of the relevant medical literature he'd done looking for reports of similar cases. Failing to find a precedent, he turned over a loose piece of paper, satisfied himself that neither side contained anything essential, and wrote down a differential diagnosis—a list of conditions that might be responsible for such devastation. It was a short list, and none of the possibilities really fit. In the end, Gottlieb confronted the only remaining possibility: he had discovered a previously unreported disease.

Gottlieb grew excited as he became convinced that the manifestations of his patients' illness represented a new, never-described disease. "The first feeling, and I can't deny it, was one of discovery," he said. He remembered thinking: *Hey, this is what you're here for. You are meant to do new things, find new things, and eureka, you're on to something that's going to further your ambitions. Your job now, Michael, is to get this into print and be credited for having discovered something new.*

The euphoria was transient, quickly replaced by a sense of helplessness. *These poor patients are wasting away in front of me. They're getting one horrible infection after another. Is this something they're going to get over spontaneously? What can I do to reverse this? Is it a temporary viral insult to the immune system? This has to be a virus. There is no other thing that could do something so awful to the immune system.*

Few young assistant professors of that era would have had the temerity to do what Gottlieb decided to do next. He cold-called Dr. Arnold Relman, the editor in chief of medicine's most prestigious publication, the *New England Journal of Medicine* (NEJM). Known to his friends as "Bud," Relman had by 1981 been the journal's editor for the first three years of what would eventually become a distinguished fourteen-year tenure. He had a reputation for not tolerating any nonsense. His career-long crusade against the rampant conflicts of interest afflicting what he dubbed "the medical-industrial complex" and his rousing jeremiads delivered from the journal's bully pulpit led more than a few of his many admirers to think of Relman as "the conscience of medicine."[9]

Despite Relman's reputation, Gottlieb said he was not afraid to pick up the phone and call him. His training at Stanford had prepared him, particularly his discussions with the intellectually imposing Henry Kaplan, who chaired the Department of Radiation Oncology. "If you could hold your own with Henry," Gottlieb reasoned, "you could have a conversation with anyone."

An associate editor, Joe Elia, answered the phone. After learning what Gottlieb was calling about, Elia said, "Why don't you speak with Bud?"[10] This was the moment Gottlieb had prepared for. He knew that he would have only one chance to impress Relman with what he'd found. Gottlieb recalled his good fortune: "I placed one phone call. I didn't play telephone tag. I spoke with a reasonable man who screened the call, and he transferred me to his boss, who was a nephrologist . . . a kidney doctor. I said, 'Here's what I have,' and he asked me a number of questions, 'Are you sure of this? Are you sure of that?' I said 'Yes. I think so.'"[11]

Gottlieb was well-organized and to the point. Only once did his enthusiasm get the better of him, when he excitedly declared that his findings might be a "bigger story than Legionnaire's disease." At the conclusion of his presentation, he got what he most wanted to hear. Relman told him, "We would be happy at some future time to receive a manuscript, but publication in the journal can take up to six months. Have you reported this to the Centers for Disease Control [CDC]?"

Gottlieb immediately recognized that in asking this question, Arnold Relman was actually advising him on how to proceed. The CDC is the U.S. governmental agency that keeps tabs on outbreaks of infectious diseases. In obliquely suggesting that he seek rapid publication in the CDC's *Morbidity and Mortality Weekly Report* (MMWR), Relman was advising Gottlieb to protect himself by accomplishing two important things: apprising physicians around the country of his concerns for the public's health and documenting his primacy as the first to recognize and describe the new syndrome. Most important, Relman assured the young physician that he would waive the "Ingelfinger rule,"[12] his predecessor's prohibition against authors discussing their findings with the media or publishing elsewhere any aspect of an investigation prior to its appearing in the NEJM.

Gottlieb followed Relman's advice. He phoned the CDC in Atlanta and was referred to Dr. Wayne Shandara, the CDC's man in Los Angeles, an Epidemic Intelligence Service officer assigned to the LA County Health Department. This was a fortunate turn of events. Gottlieb had been a fellow at Stanford and had gotten to know Shandara when the younger man was an internal medicine resident rotating through immunology.

"After a little catching up on our personal lives, I asked him whether he had been made aware of any unusual illnesses among homosexual men in Los Angeles." When Shandara said he had not, Gottlieb told him that he thought there might be a connection between gay men and an outbreak of opportunistic *Cytomegalovirus* (CMV) infection, because all of his patients either had a CMV complication, like inflammation in their retinas, or were shedding the virus in their urine.

Shandara followed up on Gottlieb's tip, speaking with a very ill young man who was an inpatient at Santa Monica Hospital, on the west side of town. After the man's death, Shandara followed the case to the sixth floor of the county health department building. There he found an isolate of CMV growing in culture that had been sampled during the patient's autopsy.

"[Wayne] decided to look into that case, and he went down to Santa Monica Hospital, and he reviewed the record," Gottlieb remembered. The next day, Shandara called. Although the case was complicated by the patient having received radiation treatment for Hodgkin's disease a decade earlier, he had otherwise had signs and symptoms similar to Gottlieb's cases.[13] Radiation might be a predisposing factor for immune deficiency, but as Gottlieb pointed out, the deceased young man was known to have been gay, and the autopsy had shown that he'd had *Pneumocystis* pneumonia.

The two young physicians wrote the MMWR case reports in Shandara's Los Angeles apartment on a hot spring day. "We wrote the cases in longhand, on Wayne's dining room table," said Gottlieb. "Wayne submitted our case reports and a brief commentary to Dick Gregg, editor of the MMWR. We had titled the report '*Pneumocystis* Pneumonia Among Homosexual Men in Los Angeles,' but the editors at the CDC abbreviated the title to '*Pneumocystis* Pneumonia—Los Angeles' and toned down the CMV association in our commentary as being too speculative." The article appeared on page 2 of the MMWR[14] behind the cover story, "Dengue Fever in American Travelers to the Caribbean." Since the CDC's Epidemic Intelligence Service did not, at the time, permit its officers to receive bylines in the MMWR, Shandara's name does not appear as an author of the article.

Following the MMWR report, the CDC sent out teams of investigators to determine whether physicians were seeing similar cases in other locales. Within weeks they discovered concentrations of patients with the same findings being cared for by physicians in New York and San Francisco. Prompted by the CDC investigators, New York dermatologist Alvin

Friedman-Kien published in MMWR a report of twenty-six gay men in New York and California who had developed an unusually aggressive version of a rare tumor,[15] Kaposi's sarcoma. The *New York Times* followed up with an article detailing the outbreak,[16] and the media drew the connection between two reports of unusual diseases occurring in homosexual men. Major news outlets, including NPR and CNN, suddenly became interested in the MMWR reports and, as Gottlieb described it, "things began to happen."

Physicians from all over the country began reporting cases to the CDC at a rate of five or six per week. "My phone started ringing with calls from doctors around the U.S. who had seen a similar case or two and now said 'Aha. There is something new going around.' They typically asked my advice on how to manage *Pneumocystis* pneumonia, which was ironic, since I was neither an infectious disease physician nor a lung doctor. I did, however, have more experience with *Pneumocystis* pneumonia than most clinicians, since before our report the pneumonia was very rare."

Encouraged by the burgeoning interest in his findings, Gottlieb set to work on the NEJM article. "To the best of my recollection," he said, "the manuscript was submitted to the journal in July. It was returned in August with comments from the experts who had reviewed the paper and made suggestions for improvements." While Gottlieb didn't allow himself to get too excited, it was beginning to look as though the NEJM, which published only a tiny fraction of the submissions it received, actually might accept his work.

"[My wife] Cindy and I sat on a blanket on the lawn beside the UCLA Sunset Canyon Recreation Center pool that August, and I revised the manuscript in longhand. I resubmitted it, and just like that, it was accepted for publication," said Gottlieb in a tone that implied, even many years later, that something magical had transpired.

Cindy Gottlieb concurred: "There is not a day that goes by that I don't think about those times. Very memorable and exciting they were!"[17]

Gottlieb and six coauthors published "*Pneumocystis carinii* Pneumonia and Mucosal *Candidiasis* in Previously Healthy Homosexual Men: Evidence for a New Severe Acquired Immunodeficiency Syndrome" in the December 10, 1981, edition of the NEJM.[18] It was the lead article. Two other papers describing patients with a similar syndrome appeared in the same issue. The lead authors were Dr. Henry Masur at Cornell University and Dr. Fred Siegal at Mount Sinai.

Gottlieb conjectured: "I suspect our article was the lead because it was the only one of the three that contained data on the cause of the immune deficiency, namely our discovery of the near absence of helper T-lymphocytes in all of our patients . . . or perhaps it was the lead because Dr. Relman remembered our telephone conversation many months before."

In the discussion section of the publication—the concluding part of a scientific article, in which reasoned speculation is permitted—Gottlieb reported that he had found *Cytomegalovirus* (CMV) in one or more body fluids of all four patients. CMV is commonly found incidentally in healthy individuals, but nearly twice as often in gays as in heterosexual men. As with *Candida* and *Pneumocystis*, however, overwhelming CMV infection causing death nearly never occurs in individuals possessing an intact immune system. Gottlieb placed his bet on a nascent strain of CMV suppressing T-lymphocyte activity as the most likely cause of the new syndrome. The authors wrote, "We acknowledge the possibility that *Cytomegalovirus* infection was a result, rather than a cause of the T-cell defect," but concluded: "At this time, *cytomegalovirus* is highly suspect in view of its prevalence among male homosexuals and its previously documented potential for immune suppression."

The isolation and culture of the human immunodeficiency virus (HIV) in 1983 from an infected lymph node by a team of French scientists would prove Gottlieb wrong. The culprit causing the syndrome turned out to be a retrovirus with the insidious capability of inserting its genetic material into the DNA of T-lymphocytes and assuming control of the host cell's metabolism to foster the proliferation of more viruses and eventually cause T-cell death.

Even so, Gottlieb's initial analysis of the deficient cellular immunity that occurs with AIDS was a tour de force. In the absence of an identifiable infectious agent, without knowing how the disease was transmitted, and with no test to determine who had the disease, Gottlieb and his coauthors made a remarkable number of correct assumptions. They had characterized an infectious disease that attacked the immune system, which was to become the most important new disease of the twentieth century and beyond.

In his online autobiography, the late John Fahey listed three reasons why AIDS was discovered at UCLA. One was the rapid appearance at the medical center of similar cases with "intractable and lethal infections." Another was his postdoctoral fellow's laboratory research, which allowed for characterization of the CD4 T-lymphocyte abnormality. Finally there was "the realization by Dr. Michael Gottlieb that this was a new disease. Deaths due to *Pneumocystis* pneumonia and other systemic infections had not been described in previously healthy men with no apparent reason for their severely damaged immune systems."[19]

His publications in the MMWR and NEJM forever anointed Gottlieb as the discoverer of AIDS. However, simply relating the story of the discovery begs the question: Why Gottlieb? Why him rather than somebody else? A simian form of immunodeficiency virus is believed to have made the leap from apes to man in central Africa in the 1930s.[20] In retrospect, there are temporally distant descriptions of patients with findings that could well have been manifestations of AIDS. Isolated medical reports suggest that AIDS may have come to the United States by the 1960s. Certainly by 1981, when Gottlieb registered his first case, other physicians were seeing patients similar to those presenting in Los Angeles. Indeed, Gottlieb recently said, "I have heard numerous stories from people who were training in New York or Miami or Pittsburgh, all of whom said they had seen cases before the *New England Journal* article came out."

So again, why was it left to Michael Gottlieb to discover AIDS? One explanation he has posed is that "unlike many physician researchers, I was always case-oriented." While many of his contemporaries focused their research on the molecular basis of immune diseases or generated reams of data to address big concepts, Gottlieb made all he could of the cases in front of him, extracting their fine details and drawing out commonalities in the manifestations of disease among patients.

Ultimately, Dr. Michael Gottlieb's discovery of AIDS and its underlying abnormality of cellular immunity was the product of happenstance and a mind willing to consider new possibilities. Unlike others who saw only what they expected to see or who tried to pigeonhole their findings into an ill-fitting, existing medical construct, Gottlieb made the necessary intellectual leap. Years later, reflecting on his discovery in an invited editorial, Gottlieb wrote, "[O]n my first day as a medical student at the University of Rochester, our class was admonished to learn to accept uncertainties in medicine. . . . [In identifying this new disease,] we did not seek to verify a particular diagnosis. We tolerated uncertainty."[21]

To this day, Gottlieb's most vivid memory of his medical career is of consulting on his first case of the new disease—patient zero, the index case of AIDS. It was only the beginning of the story. His adoption of AIDS as his life's work would soon run up against powerful individuals who had their own ideas about AIDS and those who contracted the disease.

TWO

Riding the Tiger

In the summer of 1981, when Michael Gottlieb received provisional acceptance of his article for publication in the NEJM, his academic career received a jumpstart beyond what most young physicians could imagine. In the natural course of things, Gottlieb would have turned his attention to such issues as what caused the new syndrome, how it was passed from person to person, and how to test for who was affected. These were key questions, ripe for investigation and of paramount interest to Gottlieb. However, during the weeks he spent revising the manuscript, and from its formal acceptance to the wonderment he felt as he "viewed his byline on the smooth, white [NEJM] cover,"[1] the young immunologist got bogged down in situations for which neither his education nor his experience had adequately prepared him.

Even in a large research center like UCLA, a first-year assistant professor having a research article published in the NEJM would ordinarily be a celebratory event. In fact, Gottlieb remembered a number of his colleagues being genuinely congratulatory. However, to his surprise, others seemed disdainful, even grudging of his accomplishment. He was particularly stung by his perception of the attitude of his division head, Dr. Andrew Saxon, who Gottlieb said barely mentioned the publication and seemed dismissive of his achievement. "It was as though, if I hadn't reported on AIDS, someone else would have done so soon enough," Gottlieb said.

Saxon was roughly the same age as Gottlieb, but more advanced in his research training and accomplishments. In 1978, only two years before Gottlieb arrived in Los Angeles, Saxon had been plucked from his postdoctoral research in microbiology and immunology and asked by UCLA's senior immunologist, John Fahey, to initiate a new clinical service to care for allergies and immunologic diseases. "I started this division [of Clinical

Immunology and Allergy] by myself," Saxon said proudly. "Today, people want a million-dollar endowment. I got a storage closet to sit in and a $500 loan from the hospital director, Ray Schultz. He never asked for the money back. So that was fine. I didn't have visions of grandeur."

In an interview conducted years later, Saxon's comments validated Gottlieb's perception that his chief had been disdainful of his discovery. "The virologists [who found the virus responsible for AIDS] were the really clever ones because retroviruses were new. They had to go after the problem intellectually, not just trip over something," Saxon said.[2]

In other words, Gottlieb had been lucky. He hadn't started with a hypothesis, designed and conducted experiments, and analyzed data—what Saxon considered "real" scientific investigation. The discovery of AIDS (called GRID at the time, for gay-related immune deficiency) was the product of observation. The patients had fallen into Gottlieb's lap. He had simply been alert enough to put together the pieces.

Given his chief's attitude, Gottlieb was surprised when Saxon asked to be included as an author on the NEJM manuscript. Then, as now, high-quality journals like NEJM had rules concerning what level of participation in a research study qualified an individual for authorship of a scientific article. For practical purposes, an investigator qualified for authorship if he or she had participated in the intellectual aspects of the research. Generally, this meant that the individual must have contributed substantially to the design of the study, helped with or oversaw the accrual of data, participated in the analysis of the results, helped write the manuscript, and approved the final version of the manuscript prior to submission.

Gottlieb said that Saxon invited him into his office and told him that he would ask for only one thing, and then Gottlieb could take AIDS forward on his own. Saxon wanted to be an author on the paper. "What was I going to say?" Gottlieb asked rhetorically. "He was the head of the Division of Clinical Immunology and Allergy, the man who had hired me, my immediate boss. He read the draft [of the manuscript] and suggested adding one sentence to the discussion. It goes, 'We cannot rule out the possibility that an unidentified exposure, toxin, or microbe played a role in the development of the immune deficiency in these patients.'[3] Does that one cover-your-ass statement qualify him to be an author? As things turned out, he was right."

Saxon's recollection of his contributions is quite different, but they are difficult to reconcile with the chronology and details of the individual patients. He said that he was involved beginning with the second patient to be admitted to UCLA. However, patient number two was transferred directly to the care of Dr. Gottlieb by Dr. Joel Weisman, and some of the signs and symptoms Saxon describes are ones which afflicted the first patient but not the second:

> [Someone] pointed him (the patient) out to somebody on the consult service. It may have been Mike. I don't believe it was me. But we discussed this guy. He was just a weird case. It was a weird one off. . . . Then I remember very clearly when the light bulb went on. Someone referred [another] patient to UCLA. . . . They referred him to me[4] because I had been there longer, but Michael was on the consult service. . . . So Michael and I went upstairs to, you know, "pass on the baton" . . . . And we walk in the room and he has a *Candida* granuloma[5] on his finger, a big thing, all swollen up.[6] That's what you see in children with a profound immunodeficiency. And the patient was clearly gay. He was overtly gay. He was dramatically gay. But he wasn't like the first guy. We walked out of the room and we said, "I don't know what he's got, but he's got what the other guy's got." That's when the light came on that there was more than one of these. So we discussed this, it was really exciting stuff, this new disease. So that's the paper. . . . That's how I was involved. I was actually involved intellectually.

Saxon's request wasn't the only instance of Gottlieb being pressured to include someone as an author. "We got the galleys from the journal, and I was working on them when I received a call from [my department chair] Ken Shine. He demanded that I add Robert Wolf as an author. Wolf was the intern who told [Howard] Schanker about the first patient."

Gottlieb was unaware of the deal that Schanker had cut with Wolf to include him as an author on manuscripts reporting on his patient. Wolf had somehow gotten wind that the manuscript was in progress and that his name wasn't on it. Wolf pressed Gottlieb for authorship. "He gave me the cold shoulder," Wolf said. "I was sort of ignored." Disgruntled, Wolf took his grievance to Dr. Shine. "There was no arm-twisting," he said of his meeting with the chairman. "He told me, 'I'll take care of it.'"[7]

"My team, not Wolf, ordered the immunologic tests [that revealed the CD4 T-lymphocyte deficiency]," Gottlieb said, sounding bemused. "The chairman of medicine called. Sure I added Wolf. I was new to the place. I was just trying to get along."

Shine explained his thinking in regard to what he agreed was an unusual intervention on his part: "I first became involved in this whole business because of my role as chief of medicine. I made rounds, generally weekly, to have conversations about difficult cases. Robert Wolf presented the patient's history on my rounds. . . . He was a relatively young man with multiple infections, who was clearly immunocompromised. . . .All of the usual reasons for being immunocompromised were missing." Shine continued, "I saw the manuscript for the *New England Journal* before it was printed, and Wolf's name was not on it. I remember saying [to Gottlieb], 'Why is Bob Wolf not listed as a coauthor?' Gottlieb said that he was 'just the referring physician.' But he was more than just the referring physician."

Shine felt that Gottlieb had demeaned Wolf's role.[8] He believed that Wolf's recognition of the patient's condition as something unusual enough to seek the advice of his chairman and to request a consultation by Dr. Gottlieb were significant enough actions to merit authorship. Shine recalled that the interchange with Gottlieb had annoyed him. He had felt that Wolf was not getting the kind of recognition he deserved.

Another physician in the Department of Medicine, Martin Shapiro, agreed with Shine that Wolf had played a significant enough role to qualify for authorship. "Robert Wolf was the first to realize something was going on," he said. "He had this first patient and got wind of another patient in the hospital. He talked about it to anyone who would listen. He got people interested."[9]

With the passage of nearly thirty-five years, Gottlieb has come to believe that what seemed to him at the time little more than a misunderstanding between himself and his department chair may have adversely colored their subsequent relationship and had serious consequences for his academic career. He now feels that he made a mistake about Wolf. The intern had earned authorship on the manuscript. However, he believes that Shine's memories of Wolf's role have been magnified over the years, colored by subsequent events. Had he not moved forward quickly with the arrangements for additional patients to be transferred from Dr. Weisman, called Arnold Relman, and published his series of patient case histories in the MMWR, Gottlieb argued, the NEJM article would never have happened, and the discovery of AIDS would not have occurred at UCLA.

Gottlieb rapidly ticked off the other authors whose names he had included in his final submission to the journal. He felt that Robert Schroff, Fahey's PhD postdoctoral student whose testing had identified diminished numbers of CD4 T-lymphocytes as the characteristic immunologic abnormality of AIDS, quite rightly appeared as the second author. He had added Howard Schanker to the list, mostly because he wanted to help his fellow get started in his career. "I wanted to work with him and be a good teacher. I'd had good teaching over my training, and you give back. If you've had good teaching, if you liked your role models, you want to perform up to their standards." Joel Weisman and Peng Fan, he said, had earned places by their referral of the two additional patients described in the article.

Over time, Gottlieb regretted that he had omitted from the list of authors John Fahey, the distinguished immunologist referred to in hushed tones as "King John the Immune": "I was so eager to be an independent investigator and to set myself apart from John Fahey, to get out from under his shadow, I decided to omit Fahey from the traditional post of last, or 'senior,' author."

Senior authorship is a throwback to an earlier era when even well-known researchers would add the name of their department chair or mentor to the list of authors as a matter of protocol and to ingratiate themselves with the boss. It was expected, even in the absence of "the great man's" participation in the research. In retrospect, Gottlieb felt that Fahey had earned the honorific because Schroff had been working under Fahey's tutelage. Instead, Gottlieb went along with Saxon's request that he be the senior author. "Saxon, Fahey's former fellow and my division chief," Gottlieb recalled ruefully. "Instead of advising me on what was the right thing to do, he chose to put his own name on the paper. He grabbed a piece of the glory for himself." The choice to exclude Fahey has haunted Gottlieb over the years. It was a lost opportunity to align himself with the famous immunologist and perhaps gain a valuable ally, even a mentor, who might have made a difference in his academic career.

Nothing in the tyro immunologist's life to that point had prepared him for so much ambitious grasping and interpersonal dysfunction. Michael Gottlieb was born in 1947, the second of three brothers. He was raised in Highland Park, in central New Jersey, in a house located directly across the Raritan River from Rutgers University. His mother Beatrice was the daughter of an immigrant kosher butcher. His father, Art Gottlieb, had achieved Rutgers immortality by throwing the last-minute touchdown pass in the 1938 game that beat Princeton University for the first time since Rutgers won the initial intercollegiate football game in 1869. After graduating, Art played quarterback for a season with the Buffalo Indians of the American Football League, then settled down as a high school guidance counselor and backfield coach at New Brunswick High School.[10]

Michael Gottlieb was sixteen years old when his father died at age forty-seven after a long bout with bladder cancer. The accompanying economic and emotional fallout had a profound effect on him. "My older brother had gone off to Princeton to college, a couple of years earlier, and I kind of became the senior male member of the household," he said. Given the fragility of his family situation, Gottlieb decided to live at home and commute to Rutgers.

A full scholarship eased the immediate financial strain on the household, but, Gottlieb noted, his father's death was an event that shaped how he experienced much of what happened during his life. "My dad cast a large shadow," he said. "He was a football hero who settled in his college town. When we went into town, passersby stopped and relived that touchdown pass as if it had happened the day before."

His father's death left Gottlieb with unresolved grief that took him many years to work through and influenced his decision making for decades. "Without my father, I was on my own with no mentor," he said. "I had to wing it."

The prolonged course of his father's illness gave Gottlieb a great deal of time to observe the medical profession. Gottlieb visited his father daily after school for the three months he was hospitalized. He witnessed his father's battle with pain, which the physicians dealt with by placing him on a continuous morphine drip. The medication dulled his father's discomfort but left him dazed, sluggish, and limited in his emotional range. Michael never encountered any of his father's physicians. The experience left him with a very negative impression of the practice of medicine.

"A phone call came from the surgeon who did an exploratory operation, and the surgeon said, 'He's finished.' And we'd never met the man. I remember going downstairs to the family room, opening my bar mitzvah bible, and reading the Twenty-third Psalm to get strength. I felt that medicine had let my father down . . . [a]nd let me down too . . . and so when I went to college, I studied history and American studies and hoped to be something other than a doctor."[11]

What motivated Gottlieb to reconsider his choice of career had nothing to do with his studies. His family physician was the father of one of his college classmates, who had applied to attend medical school. One day, when he was seeing the physician for a head cold, his doctor said matter-of-factly, "You know, Michael, you could go to medical school."

"I had never seriously considered medicine," said Gottlieb. "It was kind of out of my caste. I never thought that it was socially possible to go to medical school. . . . I had heard of quota systems for Jewish kids, and I knew that the kids who were premed in college were very intense. Many of the kids in college wanted it from the get-go, and here I was two years into college doing something else. I was going to be a scholar, a teacher."[12]

Gottlieb's mother had been pushing him toward medicine for some time, but it was his family physician who finally got him thinking about it. The war in Vietnam was ongoing, medical students were exempt from being drafted, and his doctor had said, "Hey, you could do this." Gottlieb took all five science courses that the medical schools required to apply for admission at one time and aced every one of them. Then he sent in some applications.

Graduating from Rutgers magna cum laude in 1969, Gottlieb had his choice of several medical schools. He decided on the University of Rochester because a Rutgers friend and classmate he admired had committed to attend, and he wanted to finally get some distance between himself and where he'd grown up. John Hanks,[13] a medical school classmate and longtime professor of surgery at the University of Virginia, reminisced about rooming with Gottlieb and several other students during their third year of medical school: "I am not surprised that he may end up as the most distinguished [alumnus] in our class. He was a thoughtful guy, dedicated early on to the idea of healing people. He was studious, conscientious, and sincerely bought into the Rochester [philosophy of] treating the whole person."

Hanks continued, "Mike and I had the same thoughts about studying. We would study as much as possible during the week, but Saturday nights were sacred. We would hit a local bar, usually the Cross Keys . . . him with Cindy and me with some floozie that didn't know any better."

Gottlieb met Cindy Wheelhouse in Rochester during his sophomore year in medical school. He had stopped by the nursing school dormitory of a woman he'd been dating for several months to say hello. Cindy and the woman had grown up together in the snowbelt hamlet of Jamestown, New York, and she was visiting for the weekend. That first meeting—when Cindy Wheelhouse briefly glided into the room fresh from a shower, her hair turban-wrapped in a white towel—failed to bring them together. However, a chance encounter at a Rochester dormitory mixer some months later did. She became a frequent visitor to the medical students' rented house on Wellington Avenue.

Cindy recalled that period of their relationship as being steeped in the atmosphere of the early 1970s: "There was one evening when we ended up in a room full of marijuana smoke after a Grateful Dead concert on campus. Afterward, I don't remember where we were, but we were walking somewhere and came upon some potted palms. We were pretty high, and John Hanks just picked up one of the palm trees and made off with it back to the house. He stole it, but I think he eventually brought it back."[14]

By his final year in medical school, Michael Gottlieb and Cindy Wheelhouse were living together in what she remembers as a reasonably comfortable duplex in Rochester's economically mixed Nineteenth Ward, on the opposite side of the Genesee River from the university. Cindy worked as a blood bank technician and was the one primarily responsible for keeping the couple financially afloat. They married in the hospital's interfaith chapel in 1974, the year following Michael's medical school graduation, during a brief midyear hiatus in his internship.

"I loved that school," Gottlieb said of the University of Rochester. "I just loved medical school. I loved clinical work, and I really hit my stride and got over—somehow got over—my previous aversion to the medical profession. . . . I was treated very well in an environment that I had some concerns about in terms of friendliness to Jewish people, and I was treated as a gentleman without any glimmer of any bias. I was in a small class of eighty students. I had a lot of attention, and people took me under their wing frequently. I had such a favorable experience in medical school that it really undid much of the damage that had been done [by the events surrounding my father's death]."

Cindy Gottlieb Sapp, now divorced from Michael and remarried, concurred: "Rochester gave Michael a prepared mind. It's where he learned whatever it was that made him what he is today."

When Gottlieb graduated from medical school in 1973, he was still undecided about what he would most enjoy doing for his career. "A plastic surgeon named Hal Bales had been grooming me to do plastics, but Hal died of an MI [a heart attack] during my internship," Gottlieb said. He had lost another mentor. Without that rudder to guide him, Gottlieb chose to continue his training at Rochester in a combined medical and surgical residency that allowed him to temporize while experiencing more advanced training in both fields.

In speaking of his eventual choice to pursue a career in internal medicine, Gottlieb said, "I remember going to see [the surgical program director] Dr. DeWeese. He was a strong, silent sort of character, a man of few words. I told him I would be going into general medicine, and he got all John Wayne on me and asked without a hint of emotion, 'Not general surgery?'"[15]

I loved surgery, but I loved medicine more." Reflecting further, he added, "I was okay as a surgeon but not the best technician. I did okay with the superficial stuff, but get me deep down in the pelvis . . ." His voice drifted off as though he were recalling an unwelcome memory.

"Even after I began training in medicine, I still couldn't decide. I liked everything," said Gottlieb. "Eventually, though, I found that I most enjoyed studying mechanisms of disease, especially feedback loops."[16] He particularly admired the Rochester immunologist John Condemi, who became his mentor. Condemi was a consummate clinician, a great diagnostician of obscure diseases, the template for the kind of physician Gottlieb wished to become. He described him as "a real Osler type," alluding to William Osler, the legendary late nineteenth- and early twentieth-century Johns Hopkins University physician. "I always hoped to be somebody who was as good as he was."

Condemi steered Gottlieb's interests toward immunology, the specialty of medicine that concerns itself with how the body discerns when it is under attack and responds to dangerous invaders like viruses, bacteria, cancer, and even its own organs when normal immune mechanisms go awry. Immunology appealed to Gottlieb because of its complexity. Moreover, it was a rapidly developing field in which an ambitious young academic physician might quickly make a name for himself. Having been an allergic child who had grown up avidly reading stories of medical detection, like Berton Roueche's *Eleven Blue Men* and Paul de Kruif's *The Microbe Hunters*, it seemed to Gottlieb that he had found in immunology a specialty that would retain his interest for a lifetime.

Condemi tried to convince Gottlieb to stay on at the University of Rochester for his fellowship. Stanford had offered him a position, and he also considered taking a fellowship at the National Institutes of Health (NIH). "Stanford is good," Gottlieb recalls Condemi saying, "but they don't have me."[17] It was a persuasive argument. Continuing to work with Condemi appealed to Gottlieb, who sorely felt the need for a sympathetic mentor. However, his attachment to Condemi and the University of Rochester was counterbalanced by several important considerations. Gottlieb had read with great interest the work of New York immunologist Robert Good, whom he described as the "dean of cellular immunologists." As opposed to humoral immunology, which deals with the role of antibodies, cellular immunology focuses on how specific cells like T-lymphocytes provide surveillance against potential threats and ward them off to preserve good health.

Cellular immunology was still in its formative years and hence a very attractive professional opportunity. Although not the only one, Stanford was a research center that had distinguished itself in this field. Moreover, the Palo Alto university had qualities that made it attractive. Gottlieb had visited his older brother Paul one summer while his brother was a postdoctoral fellow at Stanford and remembered how glowingly Paul had spoken of his time there.

For Cindy, the contrast between Rochester and Palo Alto could not have been more stark. The West Coast beckoned as something new and exotic. She recalled Stanford as everything she had hoped for: "A dream world, where everywhere you went, you could smell eucalyptus." In the end, Cindy Gottlieb had the final word. She had spent her entire life in upstate New York and was tired of the long, gray winters. She had her heart set on going west.

Gottlieb, however, faced a difficult change from the familiar environment and encouraging faces he'd grown used to during his eight years at the University of Rochester. He recalled Stanford as being highly competitive, a place where he felt people mostly looked out for themselves.

What Stanford had in abundance, however, were talented researchers doing remarkable things in immunology. For several years Gottlieb's boss, Samuel Strober, and radiation oncology's Henry Kaplan had been collaborating with Stanford's leading-edge heart transplantation program. Their goal was to safely suppress their patients' immune response enough to allow for successful bone marrow and organ transplantation using tissues and organs donated by individuals not related to the recipient. They sent Gottlieb down to UCLA for a month to learn human bone marrow transplantation techniques with Dr. Robert Gale, who was among the leaders nationally in developing the procedure. Gottlieb didn't meet Saxon or Fahey during that visit, but he kept in touch with Gale. When he was nearing the end of his fellowship, Gale let him know that Saxon was looking for a junior associate.

Saxon and Fahey offered Gottlieb their position, which included a competitive starting academic salary and a good package of resources, including $15,000 to establish a lab to continue research he'd begun during his fellowship. He also had attractive job offers from New York's Mount Sinai and Memorial Sloan Kettering Hospitals. It was an embarrassment of riches. Like so many who choose medicine as a career, Gottlieb had delayed gratification for years while watching his high school and college friends get jobs, acquire houses and cars, cloak themselves in the trappings of economic security, and put down roots. He had, by his own choice, acceded to an extended period of frugality, accepting on faith that his patience would be rewarded. In prospect, it must have looked to Gottlieb as though all the deprivation of the fifteen years since he had graduated from high school was about to pay off. Regardless of how he chose, he would soon be an assistant professor at a prestigious medical school, receiving what seemed to him a princely salary. He remembered thinking at the time, *I am going to become full professor and ultimately dean.* He was ambitious and had grand plans for his career.

The choice of which job to take was a difficult one. Both Michael and Cindy had acclimated to the West. On the other side of the country Michael's younger brother, Steven, had been diagnosed with a slowly progressive, malignant spinal tumor and was living in New Jersey. Although Gottlieb felt the pull of family and the frustration of not being able to influence the course of his brother's illness, in the end, he and Cindy chose UCLA. Cindy said, "I dug my heels in on New York. I grew up in a small town and wasn't about to join the rat race . . . having to take an elevator to my apartment and constantly on trains and buses. . . . I just didn't like the idea of going back there." In the end, Gottlieb agreed. They would stay in California.

Just a few decades since its founding, the UCLA university hospital's original red brick building was set in an oasis of green at the southern edge of the main campus, just below the big homes and winding streets of Bel Air. Gottlieb thought it a beautiful place, conducive to the long, contemplative runs he would take when he had the time. Some of the founding faculty members had come from the University of Rochester. This heritage lent UCLA a sense of familiarity, a happy reminiscence of what Gottlieb had grown used to where he'd gone to medical school. Like the hospital at the University of Rochester, the patient wings sat in the front of the main building, while the basic sciences offices and laboratories were at the back. "It was an idyllic job in an idyllic location," Gottlieb said.

Andrew Saxon was delighted with how well he had done in recruiting his new associate. Gottlieb had an unbroken record of academic successes: Phi Beta Kappa as an undergraduate, a Robert Wood Johnson Scholarship to a blue-ribbon medical school, and glowing recommendations from his supervisors at Rochester and Stanford. Saxon said, "He was bright. He was productive. He came from a good place. What more could you want? . . . He had good ideas. He was a good person. He was certainly as good as you could get, especially coming to a place where there was just me. I wasn't his boss. I was his colleague, and I was his division head."

That Andrew Saxon and his chair, Kenneth Shine, were bullish about Gottlieb's future is evident from their letter requesting the dean of the School of Medicine to appoint him an assistant professor: "As Dr. Gottlieb appears to be an excellent clinician and teacher, as well as a very promising research physician, I would enthusiastically support this appointment. . . . I fully expect that he will become a very valuable asset not only to the Division of Clinical Immunology and Allergy and the Department of Medicine but will reflect credit on the entire University of California."[18]

The Saxons helped Michael and Cindy Gottlieb find a house and get settled in the small seaside section of Los Angeles jocularly referred to as "the People's Republic of Santa Monica" for its liberal political leanings. At first the Gottliebs and Saxons had occasional dinners out together, but the time between their social outings gradually lengthened. Gottlieb's work at UCLA went very much as it had been advertised and agreed upon during his recruitment. He shared clinical responsibilities with Saxon, with whom he initially had a cordial, if not especially close, relationship.

Gottlieb believed that it was his publication of his discovery in the NEJM that put a new spin on how Saxon and others viewed him and perhaps how he saw himself. At less than eighteen months on the job, the article set the trajectory of Gottlieb's career, which outpaced most of his similarly junior colleagues. Suddenly, Gottlieb was a hot property. He was invited to speak at major conferences alongside physicians and researchers many years his senior. In short order, he sat on a panel at a major infectious disease meeting in Miami, addressed immunologists in Japan, and presented his work before the Royal Swedish Academy of Medicine.

Cindy Gottlieb often accompanied her husband during his travels. She recalled:

> There was a group of people who were regulars at the conferences. We got to know each other really well. We called ourselves the "AIDS Discovery Club." On one occasion, Michael even had tee-shirts made up with a globe and a small star for the home city of each person in the club. The shirts had "AIDS Discovery Club" written under the globe. . . . Things were mostly upbeat. It was different . . . meeting different people. . . . I met Jonas Salk at a cocktail party in Paris. A waiter offered me a canapé, and I was holding it in my hand, and I looked at it a little more carefully. I hadn't eaten meat in maybe thirty years, so I asked Dr. Salk, "This is duck, isn't it?" and started to put it down on a nearby table. He said "Allow me," then he took the duck out of my hand and popped it right into his mouth.

When he was not traveling, Gottlieb spent some of his time dealing with the press. After Gottlieb's announcement of a new disease affecting gay men, rumors were rampant. Almost anyone who could put together even scant credentials linking him or her to AIDS was on the airwaves. Public communications were rife with misinformation. Very early on, the local media recognized Gottlieb as a rational-seeming, measured resource. "Almost daily," he recalled, "I was being asked to comment by the *LA Times* when few others in authority were providing any information or guidance to the public. At first, it was mostly Harry Nelson calling me. Harry was the *Times'* well-respected science reporter. Later on, Marlene Cimons took over Harry's beat."

Cindy Gottlieb looked on as her husband became enmeshed with the local media. "He would come home and talk about what he had done and who had called him. He was very involved in the whole business . . . very taken with his new celebrity." Eventually, she said, his involvement with the media became disruptive, and it ultimately changed the nature of their relationship. "Michael became very self-absorbed in his own celebrity and how important he was. Even when he was home, he was preoccupied. He was concerned that some of the news stories weren't as flattering as he'd have liked or that they hadn't quoted exactly what he had said. He spent a lot of time on the phone. He kind of forgot he was married and had a wife." Looking back on those times, Michael Gottlieb conceded that AIDS came to dominate their lives, and the chaos it caused ultimately led to the destruction of their relationship.

Gottlieb's popularity with the press met with resentment in some quarters of the medical center, to the point that it became a distraction. Gottlieb felt that his new celebrity had been especially hard on Andy Saxon, whom he believed had been envious of all the attention he was receiving. Gottlieb said, "He was an only child, treated as brilliant his whole life, a Harvard grad. But here I was in close quarters with him. He was supposed to mentor my career development, but he was never supportive, always undermining."

Saxon denied that he or any other faculty member had felt jealous of Gottlieb. At the same time, he agreed that his mentoring of Gottlieb left much to be desired. "I wasn't supporting him fully, which is true, I was not. I don't remember anything personal or research-wise. I mean his research was HIV and mine was B-cell immunoglobulins. . . . I was well-funded throughout my career. I didn't need to work on AIDS. So my only issue was him moving off the course that was going to get him where he needed to go."

In reviewing the history of his relationship with Gottlieb, Saxon's principal complaint was that he believed Gottlieb lacked seriousness. He felt that Gottlieb was too ready to speak with the press, too eager to be accepted by the Hollywood entertainment community. "Mike got suckered by the dark side of the force," Saxon said. "That glitz of being around entertainment. . . . I mean you see it happening to people all the time. It's like a moth to light. It could happen to anybody . . . [a]nybody. Especially young people, with their attraction to the media. You know it's a very powerful attraction. He got a dose. He got a triple dose."

Saxon wasn't the only one who thought this way. "Ken Shine seemed to feel that it was unseemly for a serious academic to be speaking with the media," Gottlieb said. "Shine would stop me in a hallway and pointedly say something like, 'Mike, I opened the paper this morning and saw your name again.'[19] I would ask him whether I had said something wrong. I was very reserved around him. The media's seeking me out for a comment was symptomatic of how things were at the time. No one was providing information. Not the CDC. Not anybody."

Although Gottlieb didn't appreciate it until many years later, he now believes that Shine's sensitivity to his speaking with the media may have been primed by his simultaneously having to deal with a spate of troubles in his department that had found their way into the news. In 1980 the head of his hematology division, Dr. Martin Cline, had made headlines by performing unsuccessful gene therapy on two women with a rare blood disorder. He had performed the procedures in Italy and Israel following a university committee's refusal to allow the procedures at UCLA. The NIH revoked two of Dr. Cline's grants. At nearly the same time, procedural irregularities in the institution's bone marrow transplant program further threatened the department's research funding. The head of the Division of Oncology, Dr. David Golde, had been acquitted of a nurse's charge that he had participated in the mercy killing of a terminally ill patient.[20]

The situation came to a head one morning when a story featuring Gottlieb's comments appeared in the local newspaper and he ran into Shine entering the medical center. "Shine said to me, 'You do not speak on AIDS for UCLA. That is, you are not the official spokesman.'"

Shine remembered the incident. He said, "Mike talked to the press on a number of occasions and made it clear that he was really the GRID, and later the AIDS, guru. He was, in talking to the media, very self-promoting, and the result was a whole series of articles, magazine articles, other kinds of articles. I wasn't present when he was having his conversations with the media, but it was clear where he was coming from."

Speaking of Shine's indictment, Gottlieb said, "A major complaint about me was that I was self-promoting, but I felt the charge was unfair." He had never claimed that he was speaking on behalf of the institution. Rather, it had been the *Los Angeles Times* that had recognized him to be among a small number of experts that could provide trustworthy, accurate information. Gottlieb said that he had never once sought coverage nor initiated a news story.

"Whatever 'promotion' I engaged in, whether it was speaking to the *Los Angeles Times* or presenting my work at invited meetings of my peers in the field, it was intended, in part, to promote and add to the stature of the medical school and the hospital."

"Looking backward," Gottlieb mused, as though it were occurring to him for the first time, "my discovery of AIDS was the beginning of the end of my career at UCLA. I was not in touch with the negative ways in which administrators viewed HIV/AIDS. I was aware they did not embrace it as being their own. I think the folks running the medical center feared that people might stay away from an AIDS hospital."

It was Gottlieb's first recognition that publicity surrounding his discovery might not be welcome at UCLA. He recalled thinking: AIDS *is a disease that the institution would prefer to have been discovered elsewhere by someone, anyone, other than one of its own. That would obviate the problems associated with patients that nobody wished to care for and a disease for which there is no treatment.*

From that moment in early 1982, when his chairman warned him to be more restrained in his public pronouncements on AIDS, Gottlieb felt that the institutional leadership progressively exerted its control over him. "It felt the same as when I was a kid in fifth grade. Every day a bully used to punch me in the school yard. I don't like bullies, and that's what it felt like," he said.

Gottlieb's daily existence became an internal struggle, not just over who would speak about AIDS to the media but what resources UCLA would allot to clinicians and investigators to treat AIDS patients and conduct AIDS research. Despite his concerns that the institution's leadership was stacked against him, Gottlieb persisted in the hope that their attitudes might change. "I knew in my heart of hearts that, in the long run, the medical school would benefit from the discovery. Prestige, NIH funding and I think history, bear this out," Gottlieb said.

Gottlieb believed things might have turned out differently if he had found a mentor, a more senior individual who was sympathetic and could have advised him when there were tough decisions to be made. "I never found anyone at UCLA that I felt I could trust once the AIDS story broke. I'm not saying I was an angel. I had my rough edges. I wanted to be independent. I admit I had a tendency to joust with windmills. But I was an outsider in an inbred institution. In retrospect, John Fahey was a logical candidate, but he had been Andy Saxon's mentor. I saw him as an obstacle when I should have enlisted his help and support."

At the end of 1981 and into the ensuing year, Dr. Michael Gottlieb was riding the tiger of celebrity and media attention. Although he had no thought of jumping off, there were signs at home and at work that he should at the very least have been thinking of a strategy that would allow him to dismount without becoming the tiger's next meal. All the while, nearly unnoticed, an epidemic was brewing. Although few people appreciated that fact at the time, the evidence was indisputable. In the six months following Gottlieb's announcement of the new disease in the MMWR, health-care workers reported 270 cases. A small number of those cases involved sexually straight individuals, including two women. Astoundingly, 121 of the individuals who had contracted the disease had died.[21] Ultimately, the death rate would approach 100 percent. Not only was the disease far more prevalent than anyone had imagined, it was merciless.

THREE

Fast Times

The beginning of the AIDS epidemic in the United States coincided with intense political, religious, and cultural ferment. The 1980 presidential election of Ronald Reagan signaled a shift to social and economic conservatism. At the same moment, gay men began to emerge from the closet to openly express and exuberantly celebrate their homosexuality. In the face of the nascent AIDS epidemic, a clash of cultures was inevitable. How this played out for many gay men is encapsulated in the thoughts and experiences of Brad Hartley, a relative newcomer to Los Angeles.[1]

Gottlieb first met Hartley in 1982, three years after he had moved to Los Angeles to take a job as a marketing executive for Disney. Hartley had called Gottlieb's UCLA office for an appointment the week previously, telling the secretary that he wanted to see the doctor on a matter he described as health related.

Seeing him for the first time in clinic, Gottlieb's initial impression was that Hartley portrayed the very picture of good health. Tanned and blue-eyed, his athletic body conservatively attired in khakis, linen shirt, and unstructured tweed jacket, Hartley was strikingly handsome. He looked to Gottlieb every inch the successful twenty-nine-year-old Princeton graduate he claimed to be.

Having elicited an unremarkable clinical history devoid of recent illness and conducted a physical examination that was completely normal, Gottlieb wondered why Hartley had wanted to see him. Sitting across from his new patient and feeling that he had established good initial rapport, Gottlieb decided upon the direct approach: "So, what's really bothering you, Brad?"

Hartley hesitated, looking from side to side as though he were checking to see if there might be someone eavesdropping. "Okay. I guess I have been marking time. It's hard for me to talk about this. At this point, I guess I should either get on with it or stop wasting your time."

Gottlieb nodded encouragingly.

"I've always felt sort of like Sybil . . . you know, like I had a split personality. I enjoy being with women, but for as long as I can remember, I've been more attracted to guys. That's hard for me to admit, even to a doctor. I've always felt obliged to make an effort to portray myself as a very masculine man. When I was in college, I took women to parties even though I knew I was play-acting. . . . I played sports . . . on the rugby team. I led wilderness trips for Outward Bound. Anything I could do to make myself look as un-gay as possible.

"It worked for a while, but every few weeks I'd get the urge. When it happened, it was irresistible. I kept a motorcycle off campus, and when I got on my bike, the 'other me' took over. I would ride hell bent into the city, weaving between cars at high speed, taking turns so hard my body nearly scraped the ground. I'd go to a bar or club that had a reputation as a gay pick-up joint, someplace where I wasn't known, and become someone entirely different from who I was at Princeton."

"You'd have sex with strangers, men you met at these places," Gottlieb prompted, keeping his tone neutral and nonjudgmental.

"Yes. That was the idea. I usually ended up making it with three or four different guys," Hartley said.

"It sounds to me like you took some chances. Some of the men you met must have been pretty rough."

"At first, maybe. But once I started to meet people, not so much," Hartley said. "You have to understand how it was in New York. There were the 'haves' and the 'have nots.' I was fortunate. One night at the baths, I hooked up with an older man who had money. He liked me. He'd take me to Studio 54, Flamingo, all the top places. There was always a hubbub at the door. Big, muscled up guys asking if you were a member. Crowds of people bouncing up and down like they were on pogo sticks . . . waving to get noticed. They had zero chance of ever being allowed inside."

"Why was that?" Gottlieb interjected.

Hartley smiled. "They weren't beautiful enough. They weren't hip enough. They weren't 'known.' The whole club scene was built on the idea of exclusivity . . . who you knew."

"What was the attraction . . . just to be seen with the rich and famous?" Gottlieb asked.

"That was part of it. The places where we usually hung out were billed as dance clubs. This was the '70s. Disco was hot. Everyone thought he was John Travolta. But the dance floor wasn't where the action was. The clubs provided drugs . . . anything you wanted . . . as much as you could sniff, smoke, or stuff into a vein. Anything you wanted to do was okay. If you looked in the darker corners, people were having sex. Man-on-woman, woman-on-woman, man-on-man, daisy chains, cluster fucks . . . you name it. Not just sex. They were doing things to each other that you couldn't imagine in your wildest dreams."

"How did you feel about what was going on?" Gottlieb asked.

"Well, oh my God! I thought I had arrived! Of course it was all very exciting to me. It was later on, after I moved here, when I started to hear more about this new disease . . . GRID.[2] It scared the hell out of me."

"The bathhouses you mentioned. That must have been interesting. I've read about one called the Continental . . . where Barry Manilow would accompany Bette Midler on the piano with just a towel across his lap . . . back when they were unknowns."[3]

"I missed it. The Continental was passé by the time I started going to the baths," Hartley said. "There were two popular bathhouses in the city, the Everard and St. Mark's. The Everard was a play on the words 'ever hard.' It was like a set for a Fellini movie. The place kept trying to outdo itself, the more bizarre, the better. It was dark inside. At the top of the stairs was a very long, barely lit room. The room had four rows of beds, each with one or two men, or sometimes more than that . . . men having sex or waiting to have sex on every bed. There was a fire there one night in the late '70s. I don't think anyone was injured, but the *Times* ran a photo the next day of all these pumped up guys standing in the street wearing only bath towels."

"That must have been hilarious," Gottlieb said, smiling.

Hartley nodded with a grin. "The other place was St. Marks, further downtown. St. Marks was completely windowless. It had a restaurant, so when I went to St. Marks, I completely lost my sense of time. I'd think I had spent a couple of hours there, but when I left I'd realize that two days might have passed."

Gottlieb nodded his encouragement for Hartley to continue.

"Sometimes, I'd rent a private cabana, strip naked, and lie on the chaise. I'd leave the door open. That was the drill. Anyone passing by and looking inside understood that I was available. If they liked what they saw, they'd come in. If I liked what I saw, I'd tell them to close the door. Otherwise, I'd just ignore them, and eventually they'd catch on that I wasn't interested and leave."

"It sounds like a sort of ritual dance, where everyone knew the steps," Gottlieb said.

"The other thing about St. Marks was the steam room. It was gigantic, with a high arched ceiling. It was done up in stucco with patches of peeling paint to make the walls look distressed. The steam was so thick that you couldn't see more than a few feet. Guys would emerge from the steam for an instant and disappear just as quickly. A drop of water falling from the ceiling produced a huge echo. The effect was otherworldly."

Gottlieb had heard enough to know what he was dealing with. He decided to cut to the chase. "Exciting times. I've enjoyed hearing you talk about them. One question. Since you've been here in LA?" He left the question hanging.

"More of the same. I've gotten into bodybuilding. It helps take me out of my thoughts about GRID. I'm in with a good crowd. We all go to the gym together, work out like crazy men then hit the clubs. I'm something of a hot commodity," he said, then stopped. He appeared to Gottlieb to be genuinely embarrassed. "That came out wrong . . . I mean, you know . . . a well-educated athlete. I'm pretty affable. People are attracted to that."

"I understand. Does that bring us up to date?"

Hartley nodded.

"So how can I help you?" Gottlieb asked.

"I've been reading about GRID . . . gay-related immune deficiency, they call it."

Gottlieb nodded.

"[A]nd how you were the expert, . . . that you discovered it . . . and you're right here in Los Angeles. I felt as if I fit the profile so perfectly . . . reading about it made me want to run away and hide. But thinking I might have it and not knowing was even worse. So I made an appointment to see if you thought, you know . . . that I might have it." Hartley broke eye contact. His matter-of-fact tone failed to conceal that he was terribly anxious.

Gottlieb took his time answering. He had counseled any number of young men with similar concerns since, as Hartley had said, the media had anointed him "the expert." *Expert? Bullshit! I still have no answers for people like this. Getting right down to it, I don't know any more than this poor guy!*

"Tell me, can you recall having had an episode of what might have seemed like a bad case of the flu? Maybe a time when you had swollen glands? A fever or a rash?" Gottlieb asked.

Hartley thought for a moment. "No, I really can't. My health has been terrific."

Gottlieb considered what he'd heard. "I'm going to be honest with you. We don't know for sure how someone contracts GRID, but there's growing evidence that it is sexually transmitted. From what you've told me about your social interactions, you have reason to worry, but it's too early for me to tell if you have GRID. At this point, we just don't know enough about the disease. The only thing I can offer you is to test your T-lymphocytes."

Hartley nodded quickly. "Yes, I read a couple of articles about T-cells."

"Good, because you should know what the results might mean for you before you sign on. The test is simple enough to perform, but interpreting the results can be tricky. If the balance of suppressor and helper T-cells is abnormal, it might mean that you've been exposed to GRID, but even then, it could be something else. There are other conditions that can give a similar result. So, as crazy as it seems, it's impossible to say that you have the disease unless you actually develop an opportunistic infection. The best advice I can give you is let's test your T-cells so we can get a baseline look at your immune system. Then it's a matter of taking good care of yourself, following a healthy diet, exercising, and avoiding extremes. Be alert to the development of anything unusual and come back and see me in three months. Or sooner if you still have concerns." Gottlieb paused before asking, "So from what you've told me, you're still active on the club scene?"

Hartley nodded sheepishly. "As much sex as I've had, I figure I must have caught it from someone by now. I ask myself, 'What's a little more going to matter?'"

Hartley stood and fumbled in his jacket pocket. He withdrew a slip of newsprint and offered it to Gottlieb. "I'm not much for politics, but I saw this in the paper the other day," he said, handing it over. "It's a report of a public conversation between the president's press secretary and a reporter. I didn't know whether you'd read it or not." Hartley's expression hardened. "I was incensed! Here was this man, Speakes, who somehow has gotten himself into a position of authority, treating AIDS and being gay as though they were some kind of joke."

Hartley let the sentiment sit between them for a moment as though he were testing how Gottlieb might respond.

"I'll take a look at it," Gottlieb said, standing to shake Hartley's hand before showing him to the door. "Look, Brad," he added reassuringly. "Now you have a doctor. If you have any further concerns, or if you start to notice symptoms, call my office immediately. I promise to see you right away."

Gottlieb was outwardly calm, but in truth he was really worried for this young man, this well-educated contemporary who had so much potential for success. *If he doesn't change his ways, all that education will be for naught,* Gottlieb thought. He considered saying something but held himself in check. Gottlieb's past experiences had taught him that such drama rarely did any good. Hartley understood quite well what risks he was taking, but old habits were hard to break. Trying to force his own feelings on his patient might generate concerns about homophobia that would get in the way of Hartley trusting him should he need to seek care in the future.

Gottlieb unfolded the three-inch rectangular clipping Hartley had given him. Hartley had written the date in the upper right-hand corner: October 15, 1982. The article detailed, verbatim, an exchange that had occurred a couple of weeks earlier, during a White House press conference, between President Reagan's press secretary, Larry Speakes, and an unnamed male reporter:[4]

REPORTER: Larry, does the president have any reaction to the announcement [from] the Centers for Disease Control in Atlanta that AIDS is now an epidemic and has over 600 cases?

SPEAKES: What's AIDS?

REPORTER: Over a third of them have died. It's called "Gay Plague." (Laughter briefly interrupted, but the Reporter continued.)

REPORTER: No, it is. I mean it's a pretty serious thing that one in every three people that gets this dies. And I wonder if the President is aware of it.

SPEAKES: I don't have it, do you?

REPORTER: No, I don't. Well, I just wondered whether the President knows.

SPEAKES: How do you know? (Speakes's response evoked more laughter.)

REPORTER: In other words, the White House looks on this as a great joke.

SPEAKES: No. I don't know anything about it.

REPORTER: Does the President . . . does anyone in the White House know about this epidemic?

SPEAKES: I don't think so. I don't think there's been any . . . .

Gottlieb involuntarily cringed at the verbal jousting that Hartley had found so offensive. It was bad enough that Speakes had been so crass as to make a joke out of human misery, but to pretend he had never heard of AIDS? That was rubbing it in their faces. Gottlieb had lost interest. He skipped over a meaningless Abbott and Costello-like interchange to get to the final few lines:

SPEAKES: I thought I heard you [speaking] on the State Department over there. Why didn't you stay there?

REPORTER: Because I love you, Larry. That's why.

SPEAKES: Oh, I see. Just don't put it in those terms.

REPORTER: I retract that.

SPEAKES: I hope so.

REPORTER: It's too late.

That's the problem in a nutshell, Gottlieb thought. *The Reagan admin- istration is doing its best to ignore* AIDS. The federal agencies that should have been publicly engaged from the start were largely silent, muzzled by their fears that raising the issue might have dire consequences for their budgets. Federal research funding had been slow to materialize. The puer- ile exchange between the president's representative and the reporter was symptomatic of the administration's decision not to publicly recognize that this problem existed. Despite the fact that a growing number of straight people were coming forward with the same horrific opportunistic infections and tumors as gays, it suited the Reagan administration and its principal constituencies to continue to treat the syndrome as a "gay disease."

Gottlieb briefly contemplated his own inadvertent role in stigmatizing AIDS. His initial publications had linked the syndrome to homosexuality, because gay men were all he had seen at first. He and Bob Schroff had coined the acronym GRID. They had played with acronyms for months and couldn't come up with anything. "We had ACIDS for acquired cellu- lar immune deficiency syndrome. Well, ACIDS recalled LSD. We couldn't have that. Then, one day, we were conversing in the hallway, and out of nowhere, Schroff blurted out: 'Why don't we just call it 'GRID'—you know, gay-related immune deficiency?'" The tall Missourian's Midwest accent resounded in Gottlieb's memory. The gay community rightly objected, and the acronym had been changed to AIDS following a suggestion made at a meeting of gay community leaders with representatives of the CDC and federal bureaucrats in Washington, D.C., in 1982.[5] *Fortunately! Because, worldwide, this is not a gay epidemic,* Gottlieb thought.

To some extent the Reagan administration's exasperating policies could be attributed to bad timing. AIDS had become a lightning rod for two op- posing political movements that arose in parallel during the 1970s. One was the gay pride movement. In June 1969 New York City gays had taken to the streets after the violent, early-hours police raid of the Stonewall Inn, a Greenwich Village bar that catered to a down-and-out gay clientele.[6] Long-suppressed antagonisms between gay men and the police led to a rampage of destructive rioting. As passions slowly cooled, gay activists squared off against the civil authorities who had been marginalizing homo- sexual men for decades.

The Stonewall Inn showdown galvanized the long-suppressed gay community. June gay pride parades commemorating the Stonewall raid and involving tens of thousands of participants became commonplace in America's major cities. The parades and other public demonstrations put homosexuality in the public eye as never before. The more radical elements of the gay movement took advantage of the opportunity to feature in-your-face antics in the form of "guerrilla theater," loosely scripted to attract attention—the more outrageous and raunchier, the better. The strategy was gauged to elicit a strong reaction from those most offended by the growing gay movement's demands for guarantees of their civil rights and an end to police harassment.

Among those who felt the most threatened by the demands of the new gay activism were evangelical Christians. The 1970s witnessed an effort to blur America's traditional separation of government and religion as church leaders sought to organize their followers to promote a conservative social agenda. Among the most outspoken was the antigay activist preacher, the Reverend Jerry Falwell. Motivated by an apocalyptic vision of the havoc unchecked homosexuality might wreak on Falwell's interpretation of biblically endorsed morality, the fiery preacher gave vent to his followers' greatest fear. "The homosexuals are on the march in this country," Falwell warned. "Please remember, homosexuals do not reproduce! They recruit! And, many of them are after my children and your children."[7]

Falwell and Paul Weyrich had cofounded the Moral Majority in 1979, giving voice to the concerns of millions of socially conservative Christians. Criticized for breaching what had been the arm's-length relationship between religion and politics, Falwell responded: "The idea that religion and politics don't mix was invented by the Devil to keep Christians from running their own country. If [there is] any place in the world we need Christianity, it's in Washington. And that's why preachers long since need to get over that intimidation forced upon us by liberals, that if we mention anything about politics, we are degrading our ministry."[8]

The newly politicized religious right helped provide the swing vote that carried Ronald Reagan to the presidency. Reagan's victory gave the leaders of the evangelical Christian movement unprecedented access to the White House and the political influence to leverage governmental action on key items of their social agenda. The highly restricted flow of funds for AIDS research and a president who would not publicly acknowledge the AIDS epidemic until nearly the end of his second term strongly suggest that AIDS was among them.

However, two individuals who worked in the Reagan White House disputed that the administration ever kowtowed to a socially conservative, homophobic constituency with respect to AIDS. Donald Moran, President Reagan's executive associate director for budget and legislation in the White House from 1982 to 1985, recalled no perceptible antigay bias. "The subject [of AIDS] was beginning to migrate into the general press, so senior Reagan folk would have had some contact with the subject simply by reading the newspaper. But they wouldn't have come across it in internal White House conversations about domestic policy." Moran reasoned that Richard Schweiker (Reagan's secretary of health and human services) and those immediately under his direction would have been much more occupied with the promised reinventing of government—what he described as "bigger battles, like steering Social Security and Medicare policy." According to Moran, it wasn't to satisfy any particular constituency that the administration ignored AIDS in those early years. Rather, even if the CDC "had been screaming bloody murder" over the AIDS issue and the need for resources, their cries would have fallen on deaf ears.[9]

Moran's wife, Cynthia, concurred. As the executive assistant to Assistant Secretary of Health and Human Services Edward Brandt Jr., she sat in on the earliest policy meetings concerning AIDS. "There were many miscues, errors of judgment, plain old ignorance aplenty in those days," she said. "But in my experience, our response was not the result of a fundamental Christian bias. Not one bit."

Regardless of whether the Reagan administration was actively hostile toward homosexuals or simply neglectful, ignoring AIDS left its imprint on those at greatest risk. Brad Hartley was one of them. His narrative was a familiar one, yet unique in its own way. Like a musical rondo, the stories told by gay men of their lives in the early 1980s could present endless variations, yet they retained an essential core. Despite understanding the risks, Hartley led a sexually promiscuous life filled with possibilities for

existential harm. He had sought anonymous sex in many of the most famous gay bars, baths, and hangouts in New York and Los Angeles. He'd
summered on New York's Fire Island, the notorious sexual playground
of well-to-do gay men. Although Hartley appeared unscathed, he was a
very anxious man. The Ivy League–educated Hartley understood as well
as anyone that the laws of probability are implacable. You can beat them
for only so long.

FOUR

The Waxman Cometh

Congressman Henry Waxman had been momentarily caught off guard. He felt relaxed behind his desk in the Rayburn Congressional Office Building, and the newswoman sitting across from him had surprised him with a question for which he was unprepared: "Isn't it true that you are working on this [AIDS] issue only because you represent homosexuals?"

Waxman paused for a moment. He was unhappy about both the tone of the question and its content, and he wanted to choose his words carefully. It was true that he represented a swath of Los Angeles that included many gay constituents. They would be listening closely to how he responded. "No. But would it be so wrong if that were true? You don't question why members from Pennsylvania represent steel workers," Waxman said. "But actually, I work on this issue because it's the largest public health crisis of our time, and I chair the Subcommittee on Health [of the House Committee on Energy and Commerce]. Also, I work on this issue because I am a Jew, and I understand what it means if your society doesn't care whether you live or die."[1]

In 1982 Waxman stood alone among U.S. politicians in his understanding of the risk the Reagan administration was taking in ignoring AIDS and in his willingness to verbalize it. Because of the number and the power of those who opposed him, he knew he faced a series of battles to gain recognition of the threat AIDS posed to his country and to appropriate adequate funding to begin to seriously confront the challenge. Through his actions, he would gain the allegiance and support of AIDS physicians and scientists, Dr. Michael Gottlieb among them.

Waxman's advocacy of AIDS faced daunting political challenges. Ronald Reagan had been elected on his promise to reduce the role of the federal government. His budget director, David Stockman, was proposing deep cuts in funding for the CDC, practically halving the agency's budget. Part of the savings was to be allotted to individual states as block grants to develop their own public health capabilities. Waxman believed that proposal imperiled major public health initiatives like national surveillance of disease outbreaks and equal access to vaccinations for school-age children. Stockman also proposed a smaller but still substantial reduction in funding for the NIH.[2] The combined effect of enacting the reductions for the two agencies would be to effectively rule out any possibility of significant funding for research into the cause, transmission, and treatment of AIDS.

Even more damaging to Waxman's efforts to bring the potential lethality of an AIDS epidemic to daylight and fund AIDS research was the opposition of a small cabal of powerful conservative congressmen. Their framing of AIDS as a "gay disease" and the public opprobrium that accompanied homosexuality discouraged even those who were sympathetic to Waxman's cause from signaling their support.

Among Waxman's more vocal antagonists was William Dannemeyer, a Southern California congressman then serving the third of what eventually would stretch to eight terms in Congress. A social conservative, he strongly condemned homosexuality. He advocated criminalizing AIDS by requiring those affected to register with a government agency, subject themselves to quarantine, and in some cases undergo deportation. In 1989 Dannemeyer would embarrass himself and his colleagues by reading into the *Congressional Record* a sexually graphic speech he titled "What Homosexuals Do," in which he described gay sexual practices in clinical detail. But at the onset of the Reagan presidency, his presence on the important House Energy and Commerce, Budget, and Judicial Committees gave Dannemeyer and a handful of like-minded colleagues the influence to blunt the efforts of more moderate factions.[3] They opposed any legislation that they felt might direct funding to medical research or social services that could benefit gays. Instead, they proposed shutting down bathhouses and facilities where gay men were known to congregate and enacting social programs promoting abstinence before marriage and marital monogamy.

Waxman feared the worst for his constituents. They were in the immediate line of fire of a rapidly growing epidemic. Writing for the journal *Nature* in 1982, Michael Gottlieb coauthored an article with his UCLA colleague, oncologist Jerome Groopman, laying out the stark dimensions of a disease neither of them understood:[4]

> In January 1982 one AIDS case per day was being reported to the
>   CDC; by midyear, it was two to three cases per day.
> The CDC had received reports of AIDS from twenty-seven states and
>   eight foreign countries.
> The estimated annual death rate was 40 percent.
> Seventy percent of those presenting in 1980 were already dead.
> The CDC recently had reported a new outbreak of the disease
>   among heterosexual Haitian immigrants.
> Hemophiliacs were contracting AIDS from blood products.

Despite these ominous facts, AIDS was such an untouchable topic that Congressman Waxman was unable to generate any support for hearings in Washington, so he took his concerns about AIDS on the road. The first federal hearing on AIDS—still called GRID at the time—was held on April 13, 1982, at the Gay and Lesbian Service Center in Waxman's home district of Hollywood, California. Waxman's purposes in holding the hearing were to inform the public of the risks posed by AIDS and hopefully begin to bring together a constituency dedicated to doing something about the danger to the public's health.[5]

In spite of the curiosity of Los Angeles hosting a congressional hearing, only a single journalist sat taking notes in the front row. As Gottlieb remembers it, the crowd was small and mostly gay, perhaps just sixty to seventy people. Looking around the sparsely decorated room, he saw only a few individuals he recognized as physicians. *Epidemic? What epidemic? It's as though we're all invisible*, Gottlieb thought.

Waxman tapped on a microphone several times to call the hearing to order. He was an unlikely looking figure for the part he was about to play. Short of stature, gawky, and bucktoothed, with a wispy mustache sprawled over his upper lip, he appeared out of place standing at the head of the room . . . until he began to speak. Waxman's opening remarks were delivered with characteristic bluntness: "This horrible disease afflicts members of one of the nation's most stigmatized and discriminated-against minorities. . . . There is no doubt in my mind that if the same disease had appeared among Americans of Norwegian descent, or among tennis players, rather than among gay males, the responses of the government and the medical community would have been different."

As evidence for his assertion, Waxman compared the handling of AIDS to how authorities had managed a brief and well-contained outbreak of another newly discovered malady, Legionnaire's disease. That event had occurred a few years earlier in a Philadelphia hotel during a veterans' convention: "Legionnaire's disease affected fewer people and proved less likely to be fatal. What society judged was not the severity of the disease but the social acceptability of the individuals affected. . . . I intend to fight anyone, at any level, [who] makes public policy . . . on the basis of his or her personal prejudices regarding other people's sexual preferences or lifestyle."[6]

Other testimony followed, but at the end of the day, Waxman's opening remarks were what would stick with Gottlieb. *Here's a friend*, he thought. *He understands why no one is doing anything. The Reagan administration might want to keep* AIDS *from the headlines, but here, at least, is one government official who cares about people afflicted with* AIDS. *He understands the consequences of ignoring it, and is unafraid to speak his mind.* Waxman's hearing had been a revelation. When it came to AIDS, Washington wasn't monolithic after all.

The first person to recognize AIDS as a new and unique disease sat unrecognized in the audience throughout the hearing. He listened intently as Dr. Bruce Chabner, representing the National Cancer Institute (NCI), promised the agency would soon release $10 million to fund AIDS research. *$10 million. That's it?* Gottlieb thought. On further reflection, however, he had to admit that any NIH funding represented some progress. Seven months earlier, in September 1981, he and a number of other interested researchers had attended an invited symposium at the NCI to discuss the syndrome and consider its possible causes. Gottlieb recalled the day-long conference in the Washington, D.C., suburb of Bethesda as "very scholarly." Others found it baffling. The presentations largely focused on the form of Kaposi's sarcoma found in profusion in the "KS belt" of central Africa. That version of Kaposi's sarcoma, while more aggressive than the rare, indolent tumors of aged Ashkenazi Jews, was not associated with the opportunistic infections and other lethal manifestations of AIDS. To most of those attending, the program had held little relevance to what practitioners were witnessing in their hospitals and clinics. In summing up the meeting, Gottlieb said, "There was no sense of urgency. Few there had any frontline, firsthand experience with the patients, who were dropping like flies." There was no mention of any plans the agency might have to initiate funding investigations of the new disease.

When the hearing ended, Gottlieb introduced himself to the congressman. He also reestablished his relationship with the executive director of the Gay and Lesbian Service Center, Steve Schulte. Up to that point, Gottlieb had not significantly involved himself in the activities of the gay community. Over time, as he got to know the Iowa-born, Yale-educated Schulte, he learned a great deal about what it was like to be gay in America. Gottlieb said that his interactions with Schulte were "the beginning of my understanding, my education, in not being of that [gay] community but being allied with it, in particular, aligning ourselves with those who had contracted the disease, what [the medical missionary] Paul Farmer called 'making common cause with the sick.'"

Gottlieb was in his sophomore year as a UCLA faculty member and had settled into his work. Most people outside the mainstream of academic medicine imagine that when they visit a university-based physician for a problem with their health, the clinical care they receive is representative of how their doctor spends his working hours. They see him in a role similar to that of any doctor they might visit in a community practice, who expends nearly all of his or her efforts providing care to patients. For most, however, that is not the reality. Providing care to patients actually occupies a minority of their time on the job. This is even more the case for internal medicine subspecialists like immunologists.

For most young academic physicians, a tension develops between fulfilling their responsibilities to provide excellent clinical care and conducting their research. Hospitals tout the quality of their medical care to attract patients. Medical school deans pay lip service to the importance of clinical care, since much of the medical school's revenue derives from that activity. However, the real currency of academic advancement is success in research. Whether a young faculty member is promoted on schedule and is granted tenure depends greatly on how many articles he or she publishes, the prestige of the journals that publish them, and above all, the amount of grant money the physician attracts to the institution. In most American universities, young faculty members have six to seven years to achieve academic expectations. Failure to do so is the most common reason for the university committees that decide on faculty advancement refusing promotion and tenure. Failure to attain tenure means that the doctor will be asked to seek other employment.

In the spring of 1982 Gottlieb had only two half-day clinics in which he cared for patients. The remainder of his time was spent in his lab investigating radiotherapy as a treatment for multiple sclerosis and other autoimmune diseases, writing up his research results to submit for publication, and working on grant proposals to fund future investigations. Gottlieb initially welcomed this arrangement, since it gave him time to develop the research credentials he would need to achieve the tenured faculty position that he believed would allow him the freedom to widely explore the many important issues that already had arisen concerning AIDS.

Gottlieb's laboratory research involved irradiating the lymphoid system of a strain of white mice he had brought with him from Stanford. The idea was to weaken the immune response so that the animals would not reject the surgically transplanted skin of a strain of black mice. "They were a good strain of mice. Very gentle. There are strains of mice that when you pick them up by the tail—which is what you're supposed to do—they flip upside down and bite you. Not these mice, though." Gottlieb recalled that he had packed them for their flight from the Bay Area to Los Angeles in special boxes with plenty of slices of potatoes to eat in case the shipment was somehow delayed. Unfortunately, the animal facilities at UCLA turned out to be not sophisticated enough to support Gottlieb's immunologically compromised mice. "UCLA didn't have a pathogen-free facility, which I knew beforehand but didn't take sufficiently seriously. All the mice died of a viral gastrointestinal illness. I was very invested in my research," Gottlieb said. "I wanted to be a lab doctor and a human doctor."

It was around this time that Gottlieb encountered his first patient with AIDS, the emaciated, blonde-haired man who had inspired his inquiry into the disease. With his laboratory research in shambles, he redoubled his efforts to determine what was causing the opportunistic infections in previously healthy young men. "I wanted to flesh out the [AIDS] disease state, the manifestations, the opportunistic infections," he said. "This was a whole new area in which no one else was working. Why not dive in and run with it? And that meant studying the patients."

Pursuing clinical, rather than laboratory, research required that he devote more of his efforts to seeing patients. He found himself vying with a small cadre of clinically oriented internists for additional blocks of time when he could see patients in UCLA's outpatient facilities. In so doing, he was bucking subtle systemic pressures intended to make expanding his clinical service just difficult enough that most faculty would become disheartened and return to their laboratories. Gottlieb, however, persevered. He lobbied for and finally secured an additional clinic session. Gottlieb said of that third session, "I organized a special clinic, probably a year later, maybe late 1982 . . . what we called 'the AIDS Clinic.'" It was a clinic in which Gottlieb could take care of AIDS patients and chart the course of their problems. "And so I added another [clinic] in which to study and focus on my patients with AIDS."

Gottlieb characterized 1982–1983 as being the calm in the eye of the storm. His discovery of AIDS was no longer in the forefront of public consciousness. His superiors had accommodated themselves to the fact that Gottlieb had attained some celebrity for his initial AIDS publication and become something of a magnet for patients with the disease.

Indeed, Andrew Saxon was pleased enough with Gottlieb's performance that he asked the dean to approve a merit-based increase in Gottlieb's salary. Dated January 29, 1982, the letter lauded Gottlieb for what he had already accomplished and for his future potential.[7] "Andy [Saxon] even seemed to take pride that this [discovery of AIDS] had happened in his division," said Gottlieb. Nonetheless, Gottlieb soon found that Saxon's proximity could be uncomfortable. "Andy may have been a little resentful that AIDS hadn't occurred the year prior to my coming, when he was the only faculty member in the division seeing patients. Perhaps he might have had a chance of discovering it."

For his part, Saxon could not remember there being any tension between them until years later, when he said animosity developed in the context of Gottlieb's bid for promotion and tenure. "Early on, Mike took charge of this [AIDS], which was great, because I'm an antibody guy, and to this day I work on antibodies, B-cell immunity. . . . This was a T-cell disease, so I had no problem. I said, 'Mike, this is yours, run with it, have a ball'. . . . So Mike took charge after the first paper. . . . You'll see that I'm on the first paper and that's it. I did get very involved in the first patients because it was all new. I remember carrying biopsy specimens around, to my great fear later on, when we realized the infectious nature of this."[8]

Denying that Saxon had been more than peripherally involved with the initial AIDS cases, Gottlieb nonetheless agreed that he could have handled things better with his division chief and senior immunologist John Fahey. "I wasn't blameless. Andy was John's 'son.' Fahey had handpicked him to start the Division of Clinical Immunology and Allergies—the CIA as Andy liked to call it. He would say CIA in a dramatic tone of voice, like it was actually the Central Intelligence Agency. It was my perception that I was never going to be John's favorite, but I should have given him more of a chance to support me."

Dr. Peter Wolfe, who had been a trainee in the division and was hired into the CIA in 1984, found it difficult to imagine that Saxon recognized no tension between Gottlieb and himself. "They would have arguments," he remembered. "There wasn't much privacy." Wolfe posited that jealousy was at the root of the problem. In his mind, all the attention Gottlieb received had gone against Saxon's sense of what the order of things should be.

Wolfe acknowledged that at times Gottlieb's angry response to Saxon's manner made things worse than they might have been. "Mike had a high opinion of himself. He had a strong sense of what is right and what is wrong, and I think unlike many of us, he was unable to just let it go. If Mike hadn't been a doctor, he probably would have been a rabbi." Wolfe left UCLA after two years to go into private practice. He had quickly sensed the futility of being a clinician in an institution that he believed rewarded only laboratory research.[9]

Cindy Gottlieb was more opinionated about her former husband's colleagues: "I was really struck by how welcoming and friendly everyone was to Michael and me [when we traveled overseas]. Michael's talks were well attended and well received. His participation in meetings was always seen as an asset. All these occasions were in such stark contrast to the treatment Michael received on his own turf at UCLA."

She acknowledged that her husband's relationships at UCLA had put a lot of stress on their marriage. Singling out the more senior John Fahey, she said, "He didn't want some young whippersnapper rocking the boat. He didn't want Michael eclipsing them." With regard to Andy Saxon, she said she had been polite but remote. "I'm not the kind of person who says anything mean to anyone, but the way he treated Michael. . . . Andy was a little, despicable man."[10]

Despite the interpersonal distractions, the rapidly increasing number of patients seeking Gottlieb's care signaled the success of his AIDS clinic. The problem Gottlieb now experienced was that AIDS was such a protean disease, with manifestations that varied from patient to patient. He soon was seeing patients whose primary complaint he felt ill-equipped to handle. Of particular concern to Gottlieb were the increasing numbers of patients whose principal manifestation of AIDS was Kaposi's sarcoma or another fellow traveler of the syndrome, lymphoma. Feeling uncomfortable prescribing and administering chemotherapy, Gottlieb asked the chief of UCLA's medical oncology service, Dr. David Golde, if there might be a cancer specialist among his faculty who would be interested in managing the oncological aspects of AIDS. Golde's first thought was Dr. Jerome Groopman, who grasped the opportunity.

Jerry Groopman began his medical career at UCLA around the same time as Gottlieb but left for Harvard University's Beth Israel Hospital (now Beth Israel-Deaconess Medical Center) around 1983. Over the past two decades, he has become something of a celebrity physician for his popular books and medical essays in the *New Yorker*. Groopman and Gottlieb worked together in Gottlieb's AIDS clinic and on projects intended for publication. Gottlieb recalled one clinical trial in particular: "We traveled East and met Seth Rudnick from [the pharmaceutical company] Schering at his home in New Jersey. Together, we wrote a protocol assessing intravenous alpha interferon as a treatment for Kaposi's sarcoma. The treatment was useful in some patients, given the dearth of more effective treatments, so we published it." Gottlieb closed his eyes for just an instant. "We had some time together on that trip. We were talking, and Jerry said he thought the cause of AIDS might be a retrovirus. Jerry gravitated toward Bob Gallo at NCI. I'm not sure but that Jerry knew something about what Bob was working on.

"Eventually, Jerry and I grew apart. His Kaposi's sarcoma clinic took off. My clinic took off too, but my situation was unusual. Nationally, my subspecialty of immunology and allergy was not big into AIDS. Elsewhere, it was mostly the ID (infectious disease) people. At UCLA, the infectious disease people were my consultants. . . . They always were very suspicious of me."

The Gottliebs settled in for what both Michael and Cindy believed would be a stellar academic career at UCLA. Cindy Gottlieb recalled, "We were traveling a lot, and that was very exciting. We were pretty much in the middle of everything."

As one example, she related her impressions of a trip to Sweden during the year after Gottlieb's publication of his discovery: "My Mom's family was from Sweden, which the hosts found out before we got there, and we were welcomed into their homes for traditional Swedish meals . . . , drinks, and familiar looking holiday decorations. . . . We were invited to join a number of different groups for dinners out on the town, and even an oyster breakfast at the famous farmers' market! The handwritten recipe for *gravlax* given to me by our hostess, Inger, is the one I use to this day during the holiday season.

"We invited a lot of the people we met overseas to stay at our house or have a meal with us. One night, we invited over two Russian AIDS researchers. One was a physician, the other a PhD. I'm certain that only one of them was a real scientist, and the other was KGB. We looked out the window, and big black cars were stacked up along our street. I think that at least one of our guests was a Russian spy being watched by American CIA or FBI."

The Gottliebs undeniably enjoyed the glamour of international scientific celebrity. However, Cindy's fear of her husband's working with AIDS patients, their blood and their tissues, about which so little was known, imposed a dark side on their lives that took its toll. Cindy remembers growing increasingly disconnected from her husband during this period. "I wanted to take Michael by the hand and drag him away. We joked about ditching it all and running off to Bora Bora, going native, and never coming back."

Cindy's concerns proved prescient. She remembered that late in 1982, "a great tiredness came over me. Michael, too. He got the same thing, but his came a little later [than mine]."

Gottlieb recalled examining the patient he believed may have been responsible for transmitting the illness to him. It was a new patient he had not seen before, who presented with recent onset of the clinical manifestations of AIDS. "His name was Jack, and I was looking at the back of his throat. I was probing some filmy, nubbly-looking lymphoid aggregates—small collections of shiny, mucousy looking material that adhere to the tonsillar pillars in the back of the throat. Then, about a week later, I was overcome by this profound fatigue. It came on all of a sudden, and it felt like I had been hit by a freight train. I felt an achiness in my lymph glands . . . in the axilla [the armpit] . . . not profound but sore. Cindy had it too. I felt like I was running a low grade fever. . . . More just a sense of feeling warm. I was sure that we had gotten AIDS."

Cindy Gottlieb described the feeling that lay between them. "We were pretty sure we had it. We were dead. Michael wanted to go back east so he could die closer to his family."

Both of them stayed home from work for a week—Michael from the CIA and Cindy from her job at the blood bank—which neither of them could recall ever having happened before. "One evening, towards the end of the week, the doorbell rang," said Cindy. "When I went to the door, John Fahey was standing on the porch with a bag of groceries. I think he just wanted to see if Michael was alive, but he was concerned enough to bring us milk and a few other items." She laughed at her own black humor and at her memory of the noted immunologist standing under the porch light. In reality, both she and her husband had been grateful for Fahey's sincere concern.

The next week both Gottliebs went back to work, but little had changed in how bad they felt. It took months before the symptoms slowly resolved. Cindy remarked, "Neither of us had the energy to do anything. Then it was over, and we asked each other, 'what was that?'"

It was a question that has troubled Gottlieb since their recovery. Two years later, in 1984, Gottlieb flew to Paris. A French team at Paris's Pasteur Institute had discovered the virus that caused AIDS. Still baffled by the mysterious, mononucleosis-like illness, Gottlieb had his T-cells cultured for the presence of the virus by the future Nobel laureate who discovered it, Françoise Barré-Sinoussi.

Shortly thereafter, Gottlieb piloted Dupont's version of a marketable test kit on both himself and Cindy. To his relief, all the tests were negative. Negative for HIV. Negative for Epstein-Barr virus (which is associated with mononucleosis). Negative for *Cytomegalovirus*. "To this day, I don't know what it was, but it scared the hell out of me," said Gottlieb. "I wasn't the only one, either. Jerry Groopman came down with something. He ran a very high fever and was hospitalized for a week at UCLA. Paul Volberding had it too . . . and maybe Marcus Conant (both University of California, San Francisco AIDS doctors). I'm not sure about Conant. But it fueled my paranoia that whatever I had might return as full-blown AIDS."

The paranoia lasted well beyond the end of his physical symptoms. A few months after the illness had dissipated, Gottlieb said he suffered what he now believes were paranoid delusions. The Gottliebs had neighbors with whom they occasionally socialized. "One day, this was sometime in 1983, I think, I looked at them, and it seemed to me that they had it [AIDS] too. They looked thin and sunken, and I imagined . . . that is it looked to me that that their joints were causing them pain. Many AIDS patients get a dermatitis, so that their faces get all scaly looking. I thought they had it, but the next time I saw them, it was gone." Incredulous at this memory, Gottlieb added, "I started to see things that weren't there."

The development of delusions was a particularly ominous sign for a physician schooled as intensely in psychosomatic conditions as was Gottlieb. Brain/body interactions had been a major focus of the first years of his medical education at the University of Rochester, where psychiatry professor George Engel subjected students to biweekly viewing of films comparing a developing normal child with one afflicted with psychosomatic disease. While the physical manifestations of Gottlieb's illness eventually faded, the same could not be said of his fearful mental state.

In 1983 Jerry Groopman and Michael Gottlieb wrote a second opinion article for *Nature* that memorialized their fears and the sense of panic they perceived to be growing around them.[11] They likened the growing AIDS epidemic to William Butler Yeats's "vision of the apocalypse as an enlarging maelstrom, a widening gyre, inexorably dragging the world to destruction." They simultaneously cautioned against panic and questioned the lack of government action. At this point, the epidemic had grown to four or five cases reported to the CDC daily, reflecting an incidence that was doubling every six months. They estimated that by 1985, twenty thousand AIDS victims would be dead. Perhaps more frightening to the bureaucrats in Washington was their estimate that it would cost $50,000–$100,000 to care for each AIDS patient, despite a virtually uniform outcome of premature death.

In 1982, when Michael and Cindy fearfully suffered their mysterious and still unexplained illness, Dr. Samuel Broder was the NCI's associate director for the Clinical Oncology Program. He worked on Ward 3D in the NIH Clinical Center, the Cancer and Immunology Ward, where he treated patients, conducted clinical trials, and performed laboratory research. Broder recalled, "Sometime during the second half of 1981, after the initial CDC report, we saw a young gay man who had been admitted to our ward. He had a catastrophic immune collapse. I had never seen anything like it. I showed the patient to Tony Fauci, from infectious disease, whom I had a great deal of respect for, and he had never seen anything like it.[12]

"Everybody was terrified, but it was hard to get anybody's attention. There was an astonishing level of fear and misinformation that was the product of 'megaphone science.' Anyone with a theory could get a news story written about them, or a spot on television, and claim to know what caused it and how to treat it. People would come in and ask to have done whatever it was they'd just heard on TV. The misinformation surrounding the disease was so great, and it caused so much disruption, that some days

I didn't want to go to work. I'd never seen this level of intensity."

Broder's desire to speak out, to provide an authoritative voice during those early years of the epidemic, was somewhat hamstrung by the Reagan administration's sensitivity to AIDS and by the rules limiting what he could say as a government employee. The few times he'd inadvertently let something slip, one of his superiors had called him on the carpet. "People would call me at night, after I got home, where I could speak off the record. One night my daughter called me to come downstairs and pick up the phone. 'It's Mike Wallace,' she yelled. 'You know . . . from Sixty Minutes.' He wanted me to tell him details about the care of a particular patient. I couldn't help him with that."

The NIH Clinical Research Center is a major referral area for unusual illnesses, so Broder was not surprised by what came next. "There was an explosion of cases. . . . That's when the concerns occurred, because there still was uncertainty over how the virus—we all thought it was a virus—over how the disease was transmitted. I called everyone together and told them that anyone who wanted to could leave, and it wouldn't be a problem. I would reassign them."

In Los Angeles, Gottlieb was witnessing the same rapid escalation in the number of AIDS cases that Broder was seeing in the East. The demands of the growing epidemic kept him and the division's two clinical fellows fully occupied, but not so busy that he had forgotten, at least subconsciously, the existential scare he and Cindy had suffered. Ultimately, Gottlieb forced himself to confront the fact that while he felt fine physically, he had not healed emotionally. He decided to embark on talk therapy, primarily to address his fear of a harrowing AIDS-related death, but also to address a number of psychological issues related to his past.

Gottlieb chose as his therapist the eminent academic psychiatrist and authority on psychosomatic medicine, Herbert Weiner. He met with Weiner on a regular basis for over sixteen years, even after Weiner officially retired, until Weiner's death at age eighty in 2001. "Dr. Weiner was a much needed father figure. He worked with me . . . talked with me."

One focus of their sessions was Gottlieb's younger brother Steven, a lawyer living in New Jersey, who had been diagnosed with a moderately aggressive spinal cord tumor, a grade II astrocytoma, located in the upper neck, near where the spinal cord enters the skull. He had been treated with radiation and was doing reasonably well. However, Gottlieb knew that the long-term prognosis was dismal. "[I felt that] I hadn't done enough for Steven . . . wasn't doing enough to help my brother, even though I was orchestrating the best care I could find for him. He [Weiner] helped me to express the feelings I had about having left my mother and Steven in New Jersey and the guilt I felt over my mother having to help take care of him."

As Michael's therapy progressed, he realized that he had never adequately expressed the grief he had felt over the death of his father. Instead, he had allowed the effects of the loss to well up inside of him. "I had a great deal of anger and sadness that was never addressed and was never resolved over a period of thirty years. So when I became involved with AIDS care in 1980, I still had not dealt with the anger and sadness over losing my father at age sixteen. I had always been on the fast track in medicine, striving toward a position in academic medicine, and I had never dealt with the fundamental shaping event of my youth."

His having spent the entirety of his short career working with AIDS—a deadly condition for which there was no treatment—also had taken a toll. "I felt that I wasn't doing enough for my patients, and this led to feelings of sadness and inadequacy," Gottlieb said. "Dr. Weiner was a mentor to me. He had a broader perspective on academic medicine [than I did]. I realized through therapy and through some reading of people like [Baba] Ram Dass that there are ways that you can help as a helper, that there are ways that you help that do not have to be heroic, nor do they have to be life-saving. But being there and being knowledgeable and knowing the state of the art, being able to communicate it well to your patients, having them know that they can reach you and talk with you, that as a physician you're doing a lot even though you may not have the magic bullet or cure, that you're a helper first."

Gottlieb took to heart these revelations and implemented what therapy had taught him in his clinical practice. Sam Broder said of Gottlieb, with whom he worked on clinical trials of potential therapeutic agents during the 1980s: "There were many talented people in the field . . . and I don't want to get in trouble by singling out anyone here, because he was not alone in this regard, but Michael Gottlieb stood out. He obviously was a very gifted person."

Michael Gottlieb was among a group of leading physicians frustrated by the silence and inaction of the executive branch of the federal government, even as the AIDS epidemic grew to involve numbers of straight men, women, and even children seemingly too great to ignore. Drawing together a growing constituency urging action, Henry Waxman pieced together a coalition in support of the 1983 legislation he proposed to fund AIDS-related activities. Titled the Public Health Emergencies Act, the bill authorized the secretary of the Department of Health and Human Services to spend up to $30 million annually in support of research on emerging threats to the public's health.[13] AIDS certainly was all of that. Thirty million dollars was inconsequential when scaled against the enormity of the problem. Nonetheless, the bill's passage served notice to those who favored sweeping AIDS under the rug that their hear-no-evil, speak-no-evil philosophy was enjoying its final days.

FIVE

The Color of Money

In April 1983, as Gottlieb walked out of his office and turned toward the clinic, he heard the phone on his desk begin to ring. He considered ignoring it. He needed to check on how the allergy and immunology fellows were keeping up with the appointment schedule. If form held, the call would be from one of his several bosses wanting to caution him about some rule he'd unknowingly violated or the clinic desk telling him that his patients were beginning to back up in the waiting room.

He retraced his steps and picked up the phone. He'd been wrong on both counts. Waiting for him on the other end of the line was Dr. Marcus Conant, a Florida-born, Duke University–educated dermatologist. He had moved west after completing his training to become an assistant professor at the University of California, San Francisco. Now a senior member of the UCSF faculty, he had been among the first to connect Kaposi's sarcoma with AIDS.

The call lasted only a few minutes, but from Gottlieb's perspective, it was potentially game changing in terms of his ability to conduct AIDS research. Although he did not know it at the time, the call also would place him uncomfortably in the spotlight that accompanies administrative responsibility and exacerbate his frustrations in dealing with his medical center's attitude toward the disease he had discovered.

Conant had a connection to Willie Brown, who represented the San Francisco Bay area in the California legislature and was known to be an activist when it came to Bay Area issues. For the past several years, Brown had been the Speaker of the California State Assembly.

"Marc said that Willie Brown had managed to insert a line item in the California State budget . . . in the University of California system budget, to establish an AIDS research center in Northern California and one in Southern California."[1]

This was not the first time the flamboyant state lawmaker had stepped forward with legislation that benefited California's gay populace. Brown was an African American who had grown up during the Great Depression in a segregated town in East Texas. As a child, he had worked evenings in his family's speakeasy to help them get by. He knew what it was like to face long odds and often came down on the side of the underdog. When he wrote and pushed to passage the Consenting Adult Sex Bill, which legalized homosexuality in California, he earned the allegiance of many gay voters. In later years, Brown's open opposition to the California statute outlawing gay marriage solidified his popularity among the large numbers of gay constituents living in San Francisco.[2]

Conant wanted to know whether Gottlieb thought he could put together the Southern California center. It was the opportunity he had been waiting for. He knew that he could line up the researchers and that there was ample interest in conducting a number of projects related to AIDS. "We didn't have the money to do anything. And here was an opportunity. So I agreed to do it."[3]

All of this had occurred very quickly, based on Brown's perception of a rapidly closing opportunity to get something into the state budget before it had to be submitted in early June, so Conant told Gottlieb he would have to put something together right away.

Gottlieb called around UCLA to gauge faculty interest. He came away with about fifteen names of UCLA researchers, who several days later met up in Willie Brown's office in downtown Los Angeles. "It was quite a trek from Westwood [where UCLA was located]," he noted. "Some of us had never been downtown before. Marc Conant came down from San Francisco for the day."

Having been burnt in his handling of some previous interactions with his superiors and well aware that he was again playing with fire, Gottlieb sought to avoid any internal problems down the line. On April 28, 1983, the day before the meeting, Gottlieb had written a letter to his department chair, Kenneth Shine, to let him know what was going on: "I am writing you before the fact of a meeting at Assemblyman Willie Brown's office in L.A. . . . Briefly, the homosexual communities in San Francisco and Los Angeles have exerted effective political pressure on several legislators, which has resulted in their willingness to propose funding AIDS research

. . . as a line item in the state budget to be submitted June 4. . . . I also have informed the Dean."[4]

Gottlieb apologized to Shine for the short notice, but Speaker Brown had insisted the meeting occur immediately to meet the budget deadline. Gottlieb also listed the individuals who he expected would attend the meeting.

Dr. Shine responded on May 5, with a letter thanking Gottlieb for having let him know of the plans and for "responding so promptly and appropriately by bringing this to the Dean's attention."[5]

"I made sure to invite David Golde, who was the oncology division chief who had early on shown an interest in AIDS funding," said Gottlieb. In the end, Golde chose not to attend, but he sent cancer specialists Drs. Richard Gaynor and Ronald Mitsuyasu, the latter one of his trainees who had taken over the Kaposi's sarcoma clinic after Jerome Groopman left for Harvard.

That afternoon, at what years later Gottlieb, tongue-in-cheek, would call a "grant-writing meeting," the group split up into small teams and spread out. The irony was that the group had assembled to write the grant application for funds that were already all but assured. Gottlieb understood the need for the charade. Even though Willie Brown had gotten the line item into the budget, he wanted the academics to put down on paper how the money would be used. "He wanted us to show the UC system administrators that we had the people and the projects," said Gottlieb.

That afternoon, the writing teams outlined the projects that would comprise the beginning of the AIDS program at UCLA:

the development of a UCLA center for the study of AIDS
the investigation of tests to establish an AIDS diagnosis
studying a possible relationship between the newly discovered
    human T-cell leukemia virus and AIDS
initiating community-based AIDS educational programs to
    counteract the spread of misinformation.

If the legislative route to research funding seemed awfully easy to Gottlieb, it was for good reason. Obtaining grant funding, regardless of its source, is usually an arduous and time-consuming task. Investigators spend months preparing a grant proposal and running it past expert colleagues for mock critiques. In the end, most often with the submission deadline looming just hours ahead, they must obtain the permission of a sometimes obstinate university bureaucracy to submit the proposal to the funding agency. Here was a heretofore unheard of phenomenon: money for free.

Academic medical centers like UCLA tend to be rigidly hierarchical. Money is the mother's milk that keeps things flowing. Free money spends just as well as any other currency, but as Gottlieb learned on this occasion, not all funding sources are perceived as equal. From the perspective of the institution, grant money comes in various shades of green. While universities are grudgingly grateful for money from sources like philanthropic grants and industry funding of technical development or clinical trials, the money minted by the NIH is the true coin of the academic realm.

There are several reasons for this distinction. For one, NIH funding is highly competitive. It is hard won. A panel of experts, recruited by NIH to serve in a "study section," has judged the successful research proposals as superior to the proposals that failed to receive an award. Depending on the federal research budget, at the best of times only 10–20 percent of submitted proposals are successful. Moreover, the NIH pays a much greater amount of money than other sources in 'indirect costs" that prop up the institutional infrastructure and keep the lights on.[6] A medical school's level of NIH funding can guide perceptions of its quality and is an important input to national rankings such as those annually published by *U.S. News and World Report*. As such, medical school deans may live or die based on the ability of their faculty to obtain federal grants.

That being the case, it should not have surprised Gottlieb that the institutional response to his receiving research money in the form of a state-legislated grant was unenthusiastic. "There was a perception that because the money had been gotten politically, that it wasn't won competitively, it was somehow tainted," he said. "I had gotten the 'political grant' for the UCLA AIDS Clinical Research Center. I was appointed its director by virtue of being the principal investigator on the grant. It was for $2.9 million to be divided between UC San Francisco and UCLA. For having gotten this done, I became a target."

Despite the low regard many of Gottlieb's colleagues had for the source of funding, it bears repeating: the money was as spendable as any other money and was earmarked for research. Hence, the existence of the funds drew some attention. Gottlieb said, "Word got out about the Willie Brown funding. [The chief of the oncology service] David Golde smelled money. He hadn't wanted to take the risk of being at the grant-writing meeting, but now he wanted a piece of the action. I heard from Marcus Conant that David was pissed that Jay Levy [a UCSF virologist] had gotten $200,000. He called Marcus and threatened him. He said that he would scuttle the project, altogether, unless he got the same amount as Jay for his research."[7]

That Golde hadn't attended the grant-writing meeting in Willie Brown's office turned out to be irrelevant. "The whole thing reminded me of the Don Fanucci character in the first *Godfather* movie . . . you know, the guy who wanted a piece of everything. David smelled money . . . kind of like the Mafia. It was almost extortion—'I will derail this process unless I get my piece of the pie,'" Gottlieb said in a deep, mocking voice, dramatizing what he imagined might have transpired over the phone. "It was state money . . . it was happening at a level way above him, but we didn't take any chances. We caved to his threat, and he got his piece."

Notification from the University of California administrative offices that they were "anticipating that the augmentation request will be granted" arrived at UCLA on June 3, 1983.[8] This was the provisional notification of the availability of the state monies. One week later, Gottlieb was summoned to meet with the dean of the School of Medicine.

Gottlieb recalled, "I liked the Dean a lot . . . Dean Sherman Mellinkoff. He was very old-fashioned and very proper and a very lovely man. He called me into his office to be certain that I understood that universities do not like to be told what to study." Despite the fact that Gottlieb had given him a heads up beforehand, the dean made clear his feelings that he didn't think that Gottlieb should have gotten himself involved in state politics. In particular, he was concerned that Gottlieb had inadvertently positioned himself as representing the university.

The dean wasn't the only one who felt that Gottlieb had overstepped his bounds. Gottlieb said that Ken Shine, who would soon replace Mellinkoff as dean, stopped him in passing and asked: "Don't you think that money

should have gone to usc [the University of Southern California]?"⁹ Gottlieb
shook his head in amazement. "I thought that was ridiculous . . . not so
much from the viewpoint of what he'd said but because he would never
have said that about any other grant. usc was a private medical school, but
it operated the county hospital and was getting all the indigent patients. In
the end, Willie Brown wanted the support to go to where the disease had
been discovered and someone was pushing the research agenda."

Gottlieb conceived the ucla aids Clinical and Research Center as a
place where high-quality research would occur alongside the best available
clinical care. It would be a place where promising new treatments could be
tested to advance the science that would underpin future aids treatments.
For a while, in the excitement of getting the center off the ground, the political issues faded into the background, but there were periodic reminders
that assured Gottlieb they would never really disappear.

The legislation authorizing the awards for the ucla and ucsf centers
required that the program be overseen by the newly organized University
System-Wide Task Force on aids. The University of California administration appointed as task force chair Dr. Merle Sande, a heavyweight in
infectious disease circles from San Francisco General Hospital. A principal
function of the task force was to conduct periodic visits to the funded sites.
As center director, it was Gottlieb's responsibility to host these visits and
be sure the center personnel demonstrated that they were making progress
on the projects listed in the grant proposal. The visits were nerve-racking
affairs. Almost from the start, Sande was critical of the ucla program,
pointing out where he thought progress on the funded projects had been
below expectations. "What he noticed reflected the lack of institutional
commitment to aids in comparison with ucsf and San Francisco General,
where there was all-out mobilization," said Gottlieb. "That was his yard-
stick, but Ken Shine and the ucla administration interpreted Dr. Sande's
report as being a negative critique of my leadership."

At least one individual expressed the contrary opinion. In June 1984, after
ucla had received the task force's somewhat negative initial assessment,
David Golde wrote a letter to Sande citing what he felt were significant accomplishments that Sande had given short shrift in his site visit report. He

also took Sande to task for not taking into account that the organization had received its funding only six months previously. Finally, Golde took issue with the negative tone in the task force report concerning Michael Gottlieb's leadership: "I can state unequivocally [sic] that we have great confidence in [Dr. Gottlieb's] leadership ability, and our scientific productivity testifies to the functioning of the AIDS Center. Dr. Gottlieb already has done very well, and I believe he will grow substantially in the job in the future."[10]

Golde had copied Gottlieb on his letter to Sande. Soon thereafter, Gottlieb received a missive from Golde that strongly implied his expectation of a quid pro quo. In a letter dated June 25, 1984, which Golde labeled in capital letters, "CONFIDENTIAL," Golde revealed that his letter to Sande bore the ulterior expectation of "favored nation" status in the distribution of grant funds. That is, the chief of oncology expected that when it came time to divide up the monies, projects proposed by his division would receive preference over the proposals submitted by those who had remained silent: "As you know, I have acted vigorously and definitively in support of the UCLA AIDS Center, particularly in support of you personally as the Director. . . . I hope you have now learned whom you can trust and whom you cannot and that future resources will be allocated on the basis of contribution and productivity. . . . I have given the AIDS Center, and you personally, my support, and I request reciprocal support for the meritorious activities of my group as they relate to AIDS projects at UCLA."[11]

The criticisms the task force leveled against Gottlieb stung the young physician and would loom large in his future. For the time being, though, he had no time to waste nursing hurt feelings. Gottlieb focused his efforts on setting up the new center. "We got the money, and we organized clinics, and we began gathering data in a systematic way and bought a first generation IBM PC computer and began to freeze some specimens for further use . . . serum and specimen banking. So that's what we did with the money. [We] laid the ground work."[12]

In 1984, as the center was coming into being, the epidemic was gaining momentum. Gottlieb needed a lab technician to help keep up with the demand for testing and the growing number of specimens he was gathering from patients.

The University of California's employment system is similar to those at many other public universities. In its laudable efforts to be nonprejudicial, it leans heavily toward being bureaucratic. Finding the right employee to fill a job opening is much like joining a dating service at which the operator of the site chooses your future spouse. Individuals wishing to work on campus submit forms describing their skills and experience to a central office. The same office receives notifications from potential hirers of available positions and the set of skills required to do the work. An agency employee decides on several candidates he or she believes have the qualifications that match the demands of the job. After interviewing the candidates, the employer may either choose one of them or decline to hire any of them and receive a list of several new possibilities.

The system sometimes produces comical results, but in this case, it worked on the first try. Gottlieb interviewed Kathy Petersilie and was impressed by her enthusiasm and energy and by a midwestern work ethic he found lacking in many homegrown Californians. Petersilie had recently followed her boyfriend from Dallas to Los Angeles. She had lab tech experience, and she needed a job. Petersilie had never worked with AIDS, but Gottlieb was confident that she had the skills necessary to run his laboratory. "She was a take-charge gal," he said.

Petersilie recalled her first days working at UCLA: "It was a pretty exciting time . . . . Almost immediately after I started, there were TV cameras in the lab. Robert Gallo had just announced his discovery of the HTLV-III virus.[13] The TV stations wanted to do a background story with Michael."[14]

Over time, Gottlieb increased his reliance on Petersilie, giving her the responsibility for characterizing and managing the specimens of blood and tissue taken from AIDS Center patients wishing to enter clinical trials that allowed them access to new treatments. Petersilie's responsibilities varied according to daily needs. Broadly, however, she drew blood samples, spun down the blood cells in a centrifuge, and tested samples for the number and ratio of helper and suppressor T-lymphocytes. She kept patients' records and froze their serum for future research into better methods of diagnosing and treating AIDS. "I started the AIDS serum bank," she said. "I was [Michael's] first employee."

Looking back on that time, Petersilie was amazed at how casually she had dealt with patients' blood. "I separated blood products on the countertop. Our lab was right in the center of things, across from an elevator. I guess we reasoned that we hadn't heard of a lot of lab people coming down with AIDS. Nowadays, you couldn't get away with what we did." Even so, when the first prototype AIDS test kits became available, everyone working in the lab wanted to be tested. Fortunately all the tests were negative.

"For a while, it was just Michael and me. Later, when he had the money, he started hiring," Petersilie recalled. "He was doing stuff that was really exciting, but he was just normal. He was running in circles that you just wouldn't believe, but he was always the same." At least almost always. Petersilie knew when Gottlieb had had a particularly challenging day by what he ate. "He was a vegetarian, but every once in a while, he'd tell me he was feeling mean, and he would go eat a cheeseburger."

Gottlieb hired a physician's assistant, Larry Eppolito, to help expedite his work in the clinic. He also hired a part-time assistant, a UCLA undergraduate named Melody Houston. A nurse who lived in Glendora, about thirty miles away, volunteered on a regular basis. "She was all heart. Very compassionate," Gottlieb said.

Petersilie remembered her work as giving her a crash course in human diversity. She had been raised in Kansas and had little experience with what confronted her in her new job. A network of gay UCLA staff members had gravitated to Gottlieb's employ, including his administrative assistant, Jay Theodore, who came over from the university's office of contracts and grants.

After an initial period of acclimation, Petersilie warmed to her new social circle, and her coworkers reciprocated. She socialized with them and met their partners.

"You wouldn't believe the conversations," she said. "I was embarrassed at first. I think most people would have been embarrassed. But we were working with AIDS. You had to be able to talk with them . . . the patients too. Part of taking their clinical histories was to ask about their sexual activity. If they said they'd had 500 lovers . . . a thousand lovers, that's what we'd put down.

"I got to know some of the patients really well. They would bring their tubes of blood back to the lab and ask me to look at their T-cell activity. Then they would ask me to lie . . . to tell them their result was better than it actually was." On one occasion, a patient she had gotten to know pretty well asked Petersilie to go to a party with him as his date. "He was gay, but he didn't want anyone to know," she laughed. "I had to take off my engagement ring. I don't think we fooled anyone. All night long, I had to remind him that he wasn't supposed to be staring at the best looking guys."

Petersilie said that everything would have been perfect except for the politics at the top. She complained of silly annoyances interfering with their work, among them the tension between her boss and his immediate superior, Andy Saxon. "You couldn't miss it. Saxon's lab was next door. When there wasn't much happening, occasionally, he would come into our lab. He was really into Michael being more of a research person. Well, we didn't have time for that. But it was constant back and forth . . . raised voices. They never came to blows, but it was an unpleasant atmosphere. They weren't getting along. Dr. Saxon wasn't at all supportive."

Saxon had a way of getting under Gottlieb's skin, of making him defensive about his research, advising him to focus his efforts on more serious genres of investigation. In 1991, when queried about what he thought Saxon had been advising him to do, Gottlieb responded, "I think he meant [I should do] much more academic things, like find the gene that causes it [AIDS] . . . find the virus that does it. Or he may just have been telling me I had to publish!" Gottlieb felt that Saxon had explicitly expressed what Gottlieb perceived as an institutional bias toward laboratory research over working with patients and the development of new knowledge through the process of delivering clinical care.

In retrospect, Gottlieb noted that the study of blood and tissue specimens from AIDS patients had proven itself valuable over time in establishing a great deal of useful new knowledge. In a tone of mock self-deprecation, he said, "Well, even I know that if a serum bank had never been established either here [at UCLA] or at other places, you wouldn't know that 100 percent of patients with AIDS have antibodies to HIV. If you hadn't frozen specimens of Kaposi's sarcoma tissue from various sources, could you discover the cause of that disease? No. . . . The specimen bank eventually became a core resource of the UCLA AIDS Center."[15]

Gottlieb said, "Saxon acted as though I wasn't oriented toward publishing or interested in publishing when, actually, I was writing all the time. . . . A man named Max Dommartin, a gay man, a designer who lived on Mount Olympus in Los Angeles, gave me an early Sanyo computer because he knew I didn't have any resources and he wanted me to advance the work on AIDS. It used true floppy disks. It was huge. It took up over half the kitchen table. And I would sit in the kitchen and work on grant applications and manuscripts after I got home."

The stresses of satisfying his division head and pursuing tenure affected his personal life. "I couldn't come home from the day's pummeling and get right to work again on a manuscript or whatever without wondering if this was really worth it. I felt like I was getting battered. Cindy was very sympathetic, but there was a temptation to cash it in and go into [private] practice," he said.

For his part, Saxon could not remember any actual conflict but said he regretted any negative perceptions Gottlieb might have. "We both were young. He made mistakes, and I say that I made mistakes. I wasn't the best mentor in the world. I was a young guy doing my own stuff. If I was an old guy I would've taken him downstairs and said look, here's what's going on. I wasn't his mentor. Let's put it that way. We were about the same age, and I will say that my mistake was not having had the experience. . . . So I just let him do what he wanted to do, and I was doing what I wanted to do. I just figured that everybody would do what they wanted to do and that would be how we got there."

From her admittedly biased perspective, Kathy Petersilie felt that Saxon was letting himself off too easily. She believed "it was jealousy, pure and simple. I think Dr. Saxon was jealous of all the attention Michael was getting. It may have appeared that Michael was arrogant. He seemed to rub some people the wrong way. He was just busy and didn't have time for a lot of socializing. And then he started working with the public health people, trying to educate gay men to stay away from bathhouses and group sex, and getting them to use condoms. It really got to where he didn't have time for anything."

Although he bridled at Saxon's attitude, Gottlieb gave due consideration to what his boss had said. "I realized that the direction my discovery of AIDS had taken me had made my fellowship at Stanford irrelevant. I made an effort to retool in virology, since it was becoming clear that AIDS would be shown to be caused by a virus." He tried a number of avenues that might qualify him to work in the rapidly developing field of virology. Dr. John (Jack) Stevens, the head of the Department of Microbiology, took him on for a while, until it became clear that Gottlieb's responsibilities were too overwhelming to allow him time for in-depth study. He attempted to qualify for access to UCLA's most secure viral research facilities—the P4 biocontainment laboratories at the UCLA Cancer Center—the only place where he would be allowed to conduct research with dangerous, communicable viruses like AIDS. His goal was to start a research lab and give himself a chance to isolate the virus responsible for AIDS ahead of the French. Of these efforts, Gottlieb said, "It was very hard. I just didn't have the time."

Gottlieb had fallen prey to the mistake many talented young physicians make when their careers begin to take off. The misstep affected him earlier than the norm, but in all other respects, his failing was the same. He had an inability to say "no" to the smorgasbord of interesting opportunities that colleagues offered precisely because his work had been a success. He was simultaneously taking on ever-increasing clinical responsibilities, establishing a complex organization in the AIDS Center, and investigating and publishing on AIDS, and he had said "yes" to a heavy schedule of domestic and international travel commitments. All the while, the clock was steadily ticking away the number of days and weeks he had left to prove himself worthy of promotion to associate professor and be granted tenure. It was 1984. Four years had passed since he had joined the UCLA faculty. He still had up to three years to amass the credentials he would need to continue his academic career. He was without a mentor and was making powerful enemies within the institution.

The main point of contention between Gottlieb and the medical center leadership was Gottlieb's perception that UCLA was not investing sufficient resources in investigating AIDS and serving AIDS patients. For Gottlieb, it was an unwinnable dispute. His ethos of egalitarianism was in conflict with the reality of the medical center operating as a private hospital. Gottlieb said, "Everything we did had to be fee-for-service. They wouldn't let a patient in who couldn't pay or didn't have insurance. It was very different for

me [working with AIDS patients] than it was for people [working] at Belle-
vue [in New York] or San Francisco General [both municipal hospitals]."

According to Gottlieb, the hospital leadership had two main concerns.
For one thing, they were troubled by the fact that a great number of patients
wishing to obtain care at UCLA would have either no health insurance or
insurance with very limited coverage. The patients would either be indigent—in which case there would be no payment—or would ultimately end
up being covered by the state's underfunded Medicaid program, MediCal.
The overall effect would be that the more AIDS patients chose to receive
their care at UCLA, the greater would be the proportion of its patients who
wouldn't have good insurance. The second problem, Gottlieb speculated,
was that many of the program training directors feared that UCLA's training
programs would suffer. They reasoned that if the institution were overrun
by AIDS patients, they would have greater difficulty recruiting the best
candidates for internships and residencies.

One particular situation highlighted the disparity between Gottlieb's and
the hospital's points of view. Andrew Saxon remembered it vividly, as on
this occasion he was present. "We went to the hospital director to ask for
an AIDS ward. The hospital director was a wonderful guy, Ray Schultz. And
I went with Mike because I was the division chief. Two is better than one.
But the idea was to get a special ward. . . . And it was rejected, frankly, on
two bases: one was we didn't have specialized wards at UCLA. . . . Mainly
that was for our training programs which were supposed to be very diverse. And that was reasonable. But the other reason was—and Ray was
an honest man—he said that we didn't want [UCLA] to be identified as the
AIDS hospital. They were always fighting for their patient stream and the
revenue, and there was a clear concern about being identified with AIDS."

Ken Shine also had been involved in the decision not to establish a special ward for AIDS patients. "One area where we had tension was that San
Francisco had established an AIDS ward. I looked into that and decided that
it was not in the best interest of UCLA. We said that we were going to set up
a clinical and research team of faculty clinicians and nurses who saw these
patients, but they would not be a geographical group. And the reason for
that, in those days, was that most of the patients were very young, younger

than most of the interns taking care of them when there was only supportive therapy. And that was very challenging, and morale was very low."

Shine felt that it would have been impossible to find nurses willing to provide care in a specialized ward dedicated entirely to AIDS patients unless they were gay themselves. Without referencing Gottlieb specifically, he said, "Anytime the patients on the wards wanted something that the administration was slow to provide, that was considered homophobia, and so we decided that we would keep the patients—depending on when they were admitted—keep them in isolation, and have the ward teams come to them. And that worked quite well, so far as morale was concerned, so far as the house staff attitudes. In fact, the patients were generally okay with it. That was the only area I can think of where there was really any real tension between us and what was going on."

Gottlieb put a different spin on it: "[The institution] had aspirations for nationally regarded cardiac transplant and liver transplant programs. They feared that if we were too well-known for AIDS, that heart- and liver-transplant patients might be afraid that they would get AIDS from receiving their care at the hospital."

Gottlieb felt that he had just one powerful ally who supported what he was trying to do with AIDS at UCLA, Sheldon Andelson. Andelson was a member of the powerful Board of Regents, the governing body of the California university system. Members were appointed by the governor and approved by the state senate for their prominence, interest in higher education, and political patronage. "Sheldon was gay, a very wealthy bank president who had previously owned the 8709 Bath House near Cedars Sinai Hospital. He divested his interest in the bathhouse just after AIDS got started," Gottlieb said.

"Fortunately, I had known Sheldon for some time before he was appointed a regent. I'd see him when I visited Roger Horowitz (Mr. Andelson's half-brother), when Roger was in the hospital. I had treated Roger for *Cytomegalovirus* retinitis with the experimental drug, DHPG.[16]

"One time, Sheldon had me address the Board of Regents when they met at UCLA." Gottlieb's lips turned upward in a wry grin. "A lowly assistant professor addressing the Board of Regents. There had to be senior physicians and administrators there. It was bound to cause trouble. . . . I remember that meeting mostly because of what happened afterwards. I was privately asked a question by another Board member, Stanley Sheinbaum." Stanley Sheinbaum had married Betty Warner, the daughter of Harry Warner, who with his brothers had cofounded Warner Brothers, and was devoted to causes related to the human rights movement.

The question Sheinbaum asked Gottlieb was whether he would allow his child (if he'd had one) to go to school with a child known to have AIDS.

"I gave him the same answer I gave Joel Grey when he was preparing to star in Larry Kramer's *The Normal Heart* on Broadway. He wanted to know if he could safely kiss a man on stage. We knew the virus was present in saliva, but we didn't know back then that it wasn't transmissible by that route. I answered as I always answered in those years: 'We really don't know.'"

Despite Sheldon Andelson's support, day in and day out, the subliminal message Gottlieb received was that building an AIDS program at UCLA would be tough going: "Southern California is a very conservative place. UCLA was a very conservative institution. It's an outstanding institution, but it's a very strange mix of public and private. It's a state school, but the medical school has a huge private donor base in the entertainment industry and corporate culture. It was very conservative, and I don't think it would have been perceived very well in those communities if we were seen to be catering to the gay community.

"There's one other thing," Gottlieb added. "My impression was that the university leadership was not particularly gay-friendly. A lot of this was never stated, but a lot of it was." He recalled an exchange he'd had on one occasion with his department chairman. "Dr. Shine took me aside and said to me quite emphatically, 'We're not going to let the gay community tell us what to do. We're not going to be dictated to by the gay community.'"[17]

Shine did not remember making those statements and disagreed with Gottlieb's assessment. "Our policy was that we would take care of these patients who were suspected of having a diagnosis of AIDS. We would not turn patients away. There were some occasions when indigent patients we thought would benefit from being seen at Harbor/UCLA [a county hospital], which was our affiliate hospital down south, and occasionally patients would be referred down to Harbor, but we never turned a patient away. We saw well over 90 percent of the Kaposi's sarcoma because, as you recall, this was flagrant in that population. So the cancer center immediately set up clinics to deal with that population. And overall, we had an extremely good relationship with the gay community. They saw us as being supportive. Representatives of the gay community came to Grand Rounds and were presented as cases."

As an example of his personal efforts to engage with the gay community, Shine offered, "One of the very positive aspects was when I went on rounds, I began to shake hands with AIDS patients, and I asked how they were doing, and they would say and point into their mouth that they did not want to be intubated. Early on, the gay community was taking care of these patients, making sure they got care at home, before they were admitted, making sure that they were getting their prophylaxis (preventative treatment) for *Pneumocystis*. And they understood that there was very little to be gained from being intubated. And to me that was a wonderful development from the perspective of patient autonomy."

Despite losing his battle for a dedicated AIDS ward and the persistent feeling that he was swimming against a strong current of disapproval, Gottlieb said, "I always felt it was the right thing to do, that it was much too interesting and too exciting to let go of. And so I committed myself and tried to stay on course. I hoped that ultimately my seniors would see the merit and the benefit to the university that would accrue from having the reputation that AIDS was discovered there and being in on the ground floor of funding and other things. I just hoped that ultimately they would recognize the worth of the programs and recognize my worth."[18] Gottlieb paused for a moment, taking stock of his emotions. "I hoped that they were going to say, 'Okay, you are one of us.'"

SIX

No Love Lost

Michael Gottlieb was leading a schizophrenic existence. On the one hand, he was a junior assistant professor at a large university medical center whose leadership seemed to have mixed feelings about both AIDS and its discoverer. On the other, he was an internationally recognized and lauded researcher, welcomed and comfortable among the community of scientists that had sprung up following his recognition of AIDS.

Among those who would befriend him were two of the principals of Dr. Luc Montagnier's laboratory at the Pasteur Institute in Paris, Drs. Françoise Barre-Sinoussi and Jean-Claude Chermann. The Parisian researchers, like many others, believed a virus was responsible for AIDS.

Viruses are very small organisms, too tiny to be seen with even very high-powered light microscopes, but observable by electron microscopy. Among the simplest of life-forms, viruses can nonetheless manifest very complex interactions with their hosts. They spread through a number of different mechanisms, such as direct contact with an infected person or via aerosol droplets, as may occur with sneezing. Some viruses can live outside of cells for an extended period of time, but they are usually dormant in this circumstance and replicate only within cells.

Gottlieb first became aware of the French research team and their work in 1983, when he and Cindy attended the first major international conference of researchers investigating AIDS, AIDS-related opportunistic infections, and Kaposi's sarcoma. The meeting was held in the atmospheric lecture hall of the Castel dell'Ovo, in Naples, Italy, a historic structure that had been converted into a conference center. Gottlieb was strongly impressed by the presentation of the Pasteur Institute's David Klatzmann. Klatzmann had described a retrovirus the French researchers had cultured from a lymph node surgically removed from an AIDS patient. They named the virus "LAV."

Dr. Gottlieb was intrigued because the French had found that LAV preferentially penetrated CD4 T-lymphocytes, the very immune system cells
critical to warding off a viral attack. This explained Gottlieb's original
finding of depleted CD4 T-cells in AIDS patients. However, what he found
most interesting in the French data was a curve showing a relationship
between the level of the LAV enzyme, reverse transcriptase, and the number
of CD4 T-lymphocytes growing in cell culture.

To understand why Gottlieb found this information so compelling requires some knowledge of the life cycle of LAV. The virus attaches itself
to specific proteins found on the surface of CD4 T-lymphocytes and fuses
with the cell membrane. It injects its genetic core into the cellular "soup"
known as the cytoplasm. The virus penetrates a pore in the cell's nucleus
and activates the viral enzyme, reverse transcriptase—the enzyme measured by the French laboratory—to make a copy of its genetic material.
Finally, the virus splices the T-cell's DNA at specific locations and inserts
the copy of its own genetic code. The copied viral code takes control of
the host cell's function, in effect hijacking the machinery of the cell and
directing it to produce more viruses.[1]

So long as the T-cells are alive and LAV is multiplying within them, the
amount of viral reverse transcriptase should increase, since that enzyme
is essential to viral growth within the cells. When the T-cells die, viral
replication stops, so the enzyme level should fall precipitously. This was
precisely what Klatzmann had shown during his presentation.

That evening, as he and Cindy sipped white wine and ate *frito misto* with
new friends outdoors alongside the wharf, Gottlieb grew excited. What he
had seen and heard convinced him that the French researchers had found
it. He believed that their LAV virus was the cause of AIDS.

Not everyone was equally impressed. Virologists Barbara Weiser and
Harold Burger, a married couple working in virology at Stanford at the
time, recalled the reception the French researchers' findings received in
the United States: "There was quite a lot of prejudice against the French
group. . . . I remember that when Françoise Barré [-Sinoussi] published
her paper [describing the LAV retrovirus, in *Science*] in May 1983, it was
quite a thorough characterization of the virus. . . . One of the people in

my lab blew it off. He pooh-poohed it, saying it was only one case. It was probably a contaminant."[2]

Gottlieb had no such reservations. Impressed by what he had heard in Naples, he invited the French laboratory to present its findings at an AIDS conference he and Jerome Groopman were putting together at a ski area in Park City, Utah, for February 1984. Now considered a watershed event in the early history of AIDS research, what was initially called the UCLA Conference and later the Park City Conference brought together roughly 150 participants. It was a "who's who" of AIDS researchers. Barbara Weiser said, "Any virologist who had done any work at all in this area was trumpeting his virus as the cause [of AIDS]." She noted that Robert Gallo's lab at the NCI was particularly well represented among the attendees participating in the Park City Conference and that they were putting their considerable influence behind the NCI's virus, HTLV-1.[3] The NCI lab felt the same urgency as the other researchers in the competition to become the first to isolate the cause of AIDS.

The conference's scientific agenda was organized so as to have research presentations in the morning, allow free time for the attendees to hit the slopes in the afternoon, and have them return for a few presentations in the early evening before dinner. Harold Burger said, "At Park City, each person was to talk for twenty or thirty minutes. Gallo talked for an hour, and Max Essex, who was his collaborator, also talked for about an hour, both on HTLV-1, if I remember correctly."

Burger believed that Gallo and Essex exceeding their allotted time was not an accident. Rather, their intention was to minimize the impact of their principal competitors, the Pasteur Institute researchers, whose representative, Jean-Claude Chermann, was scheduled for the last slot of the morning session. Gallo and Essex overrunning their allotted time made a shambles of the agenda. As the designated time for adjournment came and went, some attendees grew restive and left for the slopes. According to Burger, "They cut short Jean-Claude's presentation, but he had such excellent data that [even his much shortened presentation] was more impressive for us . . . it was really pretty compelling."

In the aftermath of Park City, Gottlieb and Groopman began the task of putting together the conference proceedings. Publishing proceedings—usually comprised of short papers summarizing the presentations delivered at a conference—is a common academic practice. The intentions are to disseminate important new information to parties who either were not invited or could not be present, to archive data that other researchers might find important, and to provide an opportunity for younger and less well-known researchers to publish their work faster and with less scrutiny than is typical of peer-reviewed publications.

To facilitate their work on the proceedings, the organizers had informed the invited presenters prior to the meeting that they were responsible for submitting manuscripts that summarized their presentations. It was Gottlieb's job to edit and compile the submissions into a cogent reflection of what had transpired at the conference. Upon reading the submission he received from Robert Gallo, he found to his consternation that the manuscript contained no mention of HTLV-1, the main focus of Gallo's presentation. Rather, Gallo's contribution detailed his lab's investigation of a new virus, HTLV-III, which he now projected as the agent causing AIDS.

Gottlieb bridled at publishing what he considered to be a bait-and-switch submission. However, he said he was convinced by his coeditor, Jerome Groopman, and others he consulted to publish the article as Gallo had written it. In agreeing to do so, Gottlieb admitted that he had been "naive," but in fact there probably was more to his decision than that. Gallo was the U.S. government's lead researcher in the early years of AIDS. He had a worldwide network of collaborators and ran a large laboratory. Because he was an employee of the NCI, he was all but guaranteed uninterrupted intramural funding to underwrite his investigations. That he had enormous clout in the world of AIDS research was undoubtedly an influential factor in Gottlieb's decision to publish what Gallo had submitted.

In the wake of the Park City Conference, AIDS investigators chose sides like kids preparing to play a sandlot baseball game. What had been a simmering dispute between the American and French researchers morphed into open conflict. Weiser recalled, "There was all this politicking going around, and the politicking was actually a very big problem. . . . A lot of this was nationalism, but a lot was also about scientific pecking order. . . .

The idea that the French could beat the Americans in a high-tech scientific arena was hard to take for the American establishment."

At Gallo's suggestion, the American and French labs exchanged isolates of their respective viruses so that each could compare the other's virus to its own. Although the French researchers participated in the exchange, the prospect of sending off their isolate must have triggered a danger signal. Distrusting the Americans' intentions, they took definitive action. The next time Weiser and Burger saw Chermann was in the spring of 1984, just months after the Park City Conference. When they met his flight into Sacramento to attend yet another meeting of AIDS researchers, the first words out of his mouth were: "Whatever Gallo tries to do, we patented the [LAV] virus."[4]

Weiser understood completely why the French had taken this self-protective action. In her view, Gallo was "the sort of guy who felt that the ends justify the means. I think he did some things that were really ethically questionable and this is well documented."[5] Burger and Weiser ticked off a number of circumstances that they viewed as at least suspicious, if not worse:

Gallo had substituted the HTLV-III virus for HTLV-1 in the
    proceedings manuscript.
Researchers aligning themselves with the French were intimidated.
    In this regard, Burger cited a story told to him by a colleague,
    Dr. Murray Gardner, a well-known animal virologist at the
    University of California, Davis. Gardner told Burger that
    Gallo had urged him not to participate in a mid-1980s effort
    organized by the Pasteur Institute researchers to investigate an
    African origin of HIV. He said that Gardner had told him that
    Gallo had threatened to end Gardner's federal funding should
    he go through with the collaboration.[6]
In his capacity as a reviewer for the prestigious journal *Science*,
    Gallo had held up the publication of the French researchers'
    1983 submission, in which they described LAV and postulated
    the retrovirus as the cause of AIDS. He had done so by
    requesting an inordinate number of revisions.

Shortly following the French publication of their findings with
LAV, Gallo's lab published an unprecedented four articles in
a single issue of *Science*, detailing the case for HTLV-III. The
publications described the development of a cell line they had
used to culture their virus. Burger believed that the cell line
had been derived from cells originally cultured in a nearby NCI
laboratory.

Most damning in the eyes of Burger and Weiser, however, was that Gallo
had turned over the assessment of the French isolate he had received from
Barré-Sinoussi to a member of his laboratory, Dr. Mikulas Popovic. Popovic
was to conduct the genetic sequencing that would determine the similarity
of the French LAV to Gallo's HTLV-III. When concerns arose over the nearly
identical genetic sequences of the two viruses, and the NIH initiated an
investigation, Popovic admitted that he might have combined a number
of different isolates into a sort of viral stew. He further stipulated that one
of the ingredients of the *gemisch* might well have been the cell culture sent
by the researchers at the Pasteur Institute.

Harold Burger was incredulous. "You don't have to be a microbiologist
to know that this is not cooking. This is supposed to be science. You don't
just add it to the pot and see what comes out. I mean this is elementary.
They violated that elementary principal. He threw in a mixture of different
sources."

Popovic's analysis showed a less than 1 percent difference in the genetics
of the Pasteur Institute's LAV and Gallo's HTLV-III. What makes this such
a remarkable (and questionable) result is that HIV is a highly mutable virus,
a fact that continues to bedevil investigators seeking to invent an effective
vaccine even today. Burger asserted that just the passage of HIV from one
person to another results in an average genetic difference of approximately
8 percent. This was the level of variation Dr. Jay Levy's laboratory at the
University of California San Francisco found between his own independent
isolate, named ARV, and the French LAV.[7] The NCI laboratory's finding only
a 1 percent divergence in the genetics between LAV and HTLV-III made it
exceedingly likely that not only were the two viruses one and the same,
but that they had been cultured from the same source.

Despite the similarity of the NCI and the Pasteur Institute viruses, in 1984 the U.S. Patent Office granted a patent to the NCI, on behalf of Dr. Gallo, for a diagnostic test for HIV based on his culturing of HTLV-III. As HTLV-III was identical to LAV, as shown by the Gallo lab's own analysis, the Pasteur Institute sued Dr. Gallo and the U.S. government for infringement on their previously patented intellectual property. There followed several years of litigation that enveloped not only the lawyers for the two parties but also the scientists.

"I tried as much as I could to stay away from this," said Barré-Sinoussi. "Like all the people involved, I had to be heard by lawyers."[8] In the end, the French and U.S. governments agreed to split use fees and other revenues derived from HIV.

The conflict between the two research groups extended to their disagreeing over what the virus should be named. Barbara Weiser recalled that until 1987 she and her husband took no chances, referring to the virus as LAV/HTLV-III. Beginning in 1987, following the recommendation of the International Committee on the Taxonomy of Viruses, the AIDS virus was uniformly called HIV.[9]

A nearly book-length article by John Crewdson, appearing in the *Chicago Tribune* on November 19, 1989,[10] tracked these and other concerns over how Robert Gallo had comported himself during his research on AIDS. Spurred by Crewdson's findings, a series of three high-level federal research investigations, plus a senatorial inquiry led by Senator Charles Grassley (R-IA), uncovered a number of irregularities in the procedures employed by Gallo's laboratory. Ultimately, however, Gallo was absolved of significant wrongdoing. He left the NCI in 1996 to become the director of the Institute of Human Virology at the University of Maryland.

Anders Vahlne, a professor of microbiology at Sweden's Karolinska Institute, offered an alternative view to Crewdson's of this antagonistic history. In the wake of the 2008 Nobel Prize being conferred on Luc Montagnier and Françoise Barré-Sinoussi for their discovery of HIV and on Harald zur Hausen for his discovery of the human papilloma virus (HPV), Vahlne wrote: "Unfortunately, the omission of the American scientist Robert C. Gallo from the 2008 Nobel Prize in Medicine or Physiology for the discovery of HIV by many has been viewed as a final scientific verdict handed down by the Nobel Committee of the Karolinska Institute on an old controversy between the Institute Pasteur and NIH and that previous settlements were for political reasons only."[11]

Although Vahlne did not specifically single out Crewdson in the following excerpt, he made clear where his sentiments lay: "Also, the decision to omit Gallo has resulted in the resurrection of false allegations in the media that Gallo and coworkers at NIH had rediscovered or even stolen the French HIV isolate previously sent to them from the Pasteur Institute."

Vahlne asserted that he "painstakingly and thoroughly [went] through all of the literature related to the discovery of HIV." His conclusion: "There is no doubt or controversy about the fact that the French group was first to isolate this new virus. This is what the Nobel committee chose to award."

Case closed. Even so, Vahlne noted that the French researchers substantially benefited from the work of the Gallo laboratory:

Montagnier indirectly got the idea for isolating a retrovirus
    from the Gallo laboratory.
The French used protocols for virus isolation and reverse
    transcriptase analysis from Gallo's work with HTLV-1.
Barré-Sinoussi had spent a sabbatical in Gallo's laboratory,
    where she learned to culture lymphocytes.
Gallo was the first to validate that the French LAV was the
    cause of AIDS.
Gallo was the first to develop a blood test for screening
    blood donors for HIV infection, thereby saving hundreds
    of thousands of lives.

Vahlne further concluded that as Gallo and his laboratory had been scrutinized for almost five years by three different NIH investigations and emerged without sufficient evidence to sustain the charges of scientific misconduct, perpetuation of allegations to the contrary should be laid to rest.

The deliberations leading to the awarding of a Nobel Prize are sealed for fifty years, leaving only speculation concerning what considerations led to the selection of the 2008 Nobel laureates. Despite Vahlne's assertions, it is difficult to imagine that the members of the Nobel Committee for Physiology or Medicine completely ignored the controversy surrounding Robert Gallo in their deliberations.[12] The history of the Nobel Prize is rife with controversial choices, and the Nobel Assembly, which makes the final decision on the prize, is notoriously cautious about knowingly choosing a laureate whose work might later be shown to be suspect.

The process of determining who will be awarded a prize for medicine or physiology begins with the Nobel Medicine or Physiology Committee. The committee receives and considers nominations made earlier in the year by qualified nominators. These include members of the Nobel Assembly, Swedish and foreign members of the Royal Swedish Academy of Sciences, Nobel laureates in physiology or medicine and chemistry, professors of medicine at universities in Scandinavia, invited nominators from no fewer than six universities chosen by the assembly, ad hoc nominators invited by the assembly, and the members of the committee.

The committee makes a recommendation to the Nobel Assembly, which most often, but not always, accepts the recommendation in making the final decision. As shown in this instance, how the committee chooses to frame the reason for awarding a prize can have much to do with who among the nominees eventually is chosen. In the case of the 2008 Nobel Prize for Medicine or Physiology, the decision to reward the discovery of important human viruses dictated the outcome. As Vahlne noted, "This is what the Nobel committee chose to award."

Among the rules governing the awarding of Nobel Prizes is a stricture prohibiting more than three individuals sharing a prize in a given year.[13] Once it was decided that the prize would go to the discoverers of human viruses, there could be no further scientific arguments in favor of Gallo. Everyone agreed that the French had primacy. Moreover, in selecting zur Hausen to share the prize, the assembly filled out its maximum complement of three laureates, minimizing any carping that might have developed over its exclusion of Robert Gallo.

Was Michael Gottlieb ever considered for the Nobel Prize? Again, in this case, the framing of the prize was everything. If the Medicine or Physiology Committee had chosen to focus its nomination exclusively on AIDS and who had made key contributions to the early history of the epidemic, rather than to the isolation of viruses, it is not beyond imagination that he might have received some consideration. In fact, there is evidence that the committee did explore the possibility of an "AIDS prize," at least early in the process. During a 2010 symposium Gottlieb attended at the University of California, Davis, the former dean of the university's School of Public Health, Dr. Roger Detels, told Gottlieb that the Nobel committee had inquired about him. Moreover, Andrew Saxon asserted that he'd also had a conversation with representatives of the Nobel committee. As committee members undoubtedly are accustomed to hearing effusive praise from the colleagues of potential nominees, they must have been astounded when Saxon advised them to address their attentions to those who had identified HIV as the causative agent.[14]

On the evening of December 10, 2008, Professors Montagnier, Barré-Sinoussi, and zur Hausen sat in the front row of Stockholm's crowded Concert Hall, alongside a stage lined with red roses and white carnations. Adhering to the directions provided every male laureate since the first prizes were awarded in 1901, the men sported formal, cutaway black jackets, matching trousers, a white formal shirt, and white bowtie. Françoise Barré-Sinoussi received her award attired in an unadorned floor-length black gown, set off by strands of small diamonds at her ears and throat.[15]

Karolinska Institute professor Jan Andersson introduced the laureates in physiology or medicine: "Dear Laureates. On behalf of the Nobel Assembly at the Karolinska Institute, it is my pleasure and privilege to express our warmest congratulations and deepest admiration as I now ask you to step forward to receive your medal and diploma from the hands of His Majesty the King."

Tall and thin, his hair swept back along the sides, King Carl Gustaf stood beside his elegantly dressed queen of thirty-two years to greet each laureate in turn and present him or her with the medal and diploma symbolic of the Nobel Prize. Not mentioned in the course of the ceremony was the substantial monetary award that also is a part of the prize (the 2015 value of the 2008 prize is $1,163,030). The Nobel Assembly granted a quarter share each to Drs. Montagnier and Barré-Sinoussi, and a half share to Harald zur Hausen.[16]

After the ceremony, the laureates followed the royal family to the Blue Hall of nearby Stockholm City Hall. The banquet room was filled with long parallel rows of linen-covered tables for a candlelit dinner set for thirteen hundred people. Each year the chefs, honored by the selection, do their best to outdo those who have preceded them. The menu for 2008 featured a mélange of meats and seafood individually paired with accompanying glasses of wine, and for dessert, a pear poached in burgundy, ensconced in a puddle of whipped cream.[17] Replete with music, toasts, speeches, and the traditions that had developed since the awarding of the first prizes in 1901, the event extended well past midnight.

The celebratory evening capped an exhausting week during which Barré-Sinoussi delivered the traditional Nobel lecture. Three days earlier, on December 7, she had stood alone at the base of a spare, steeply canted, wood-lined amphitheater in the Karolinska Institute. Only a small arrangement of flowers to the right of the podium adorned the stage.

Looking stylish in a pink and gray print dress and wearing rimless glasses, her short, silver-streaked hair rimming her face, Barré-Sinoussi presented in French-tinted English a forty-five-minute lecture, "HIV: A Discovery Opening the Road to Novel Scientific Knowledge and Global Health Improvement." Her presentation emphasized not only her team's discovery of HIV, but also the implications of the discovery for improving scientific knowledge and ultimately a hoped-for improvement in global health.

In the first minutes of her lecture, without specifically mentioning the discovery of AIDS, she gave a nod to the power of medical observation in generating the hypotheses that led to their uncovering HIV as the infectious agent. Her only mention of Robert Gallo was when she noted: "In 1984, R. Gallo and colleagues and J. Levy and coworkers published reports confirming the identification of the virus shown to cause AIDS."[18]

During the lead-up to the presentation of the 2008 awards, the assembly's selections for the Medicine or Physiology Prize had been a topic of considerable media interest. Ake Spross, a reporter for the Swedish daily *Upsala Nya Tidning*, e-mailed Michael Gottlieb to get his perspective. "Did they get it right?" he wanted to know.

Gottlieb's response was, "Unquestionably correct. Barré-Sinoussi and colleagues set out to find the cause of AIDS and designed experiments based on the observed depletion of CD-4 T-cells in AIDS patients. At the time, a viral cause was but one of many hypotheses. They found their virus (LAV) within two years of the identification of the new disease, a remarkable feat. . . . The dramatically improved prognosis for HIV today is due in large part to the rapid identification of the causative agent. As an aside, I first learned of their work in a 1983 conference in Naples, Italy. . . . When I saw their data and heard the story I got goose bumps. I remember the moment when I said to myself 'They've got it!'"[19]

In a 2014 interview, Barré-Sinoussi said that at the moment of discovery, she never imagined that she would have such an experience. It never occurred to her how what she and her team had set into motion might turn out. "That it would change the rest of my life? Certainly not. I remember I told my husband, who wasn't very happy because I wasn't very often at home, 'Don't worry it's just, you know, for one, two years maybe, and then it will be over.'"[20]

Barré-Sinoussi's thoughts about the events surrounding that period and her feelings toward Robert Gallo are surprising. In the same 2014 interview, she said that she had kept in close contact with Dr. Gallo and that they had jointly organized a retrospective conference on AIDS at the Pasteur Institute in 2011. "For me it's a Nobel Prize for all the community of people that has been working [on it]. It's not my prize, it's our prize," she said.[21]

SEVEN

The Power of Denial

"Hey, Doc!"

Gottlieb hopped from the asphalt onto the sidewalk just after the light had turned green, looking behind him as traffic started to move on Santa Monica Boulevard. There was something familiar about the tall, white-clad figure jogging toward him waving a tennis racket in his left hand while his right warded off the cars edging toward him with a classic stiff-arm.

Still uncertain about whom he was greeting, Gottlieb accepted the man's right hand and shook it.

"Doc! Good to see you. Brad . . . Brad Hartley," the man said, with a questioning upward lilt. "I'm one of your patients. I saw you in your office a couple of years ago, back in 1982. You ran a few tests that came back okay."

"Of course," Gottlieb said. He stretched his memory trying to recall something of Hartley's visit. "How are you?"

"I'm doing well. Really well! Thanks for asking."

"Doc, I don't mean to be a nuisance. If it's a problem, just say so, and we'll leave things as they are, just an unexpected chance to say 'hello.' But when I saw you walking across the street, it occurred to me that I was going to give you a call anyways. I've been traveling recently, back to my old stomping grounds in New York, and there are a few things I need to get off my chest. Do you have time to let me buy you a cup of coffee?"

Gottlieb hesitated a moment, considering what he had scheduled for the afternoon.

Seeing Gottlieb's uncertainty, Hartley said, "I understand Doc. I don't know why I asked. Anyone can see that you're on your way somewhere." Hartley once again held out his hand. "Great seeing you. We'll talk soon."

Over the years of his training and clinical practice, Gottlieb had developed something of a sixth sense. He usually could recognize when something important was being left unsaid. Despite Hartley's avowal of good health, there was something in the man's voice that put Gottlieb on the alert. "Sure. I have a few minutes if it's something important," he said.

"That's terrific of you, Doc," Hartley said a little too quickly, as though he were afraid Gottlieb might change his mind. "There's a small coffee shop just down the block. If you like your java dark and thick, this is your kind of place."

Gottlieb smiled and followed Hartley around the corner to a small storefront. Hartley held open the door and pointed to a table in the back corner of a cramped, dimly lit space. The shop was dominated by an oversized Italian coffeemaker behind a counter that ran along one side of the room. A young man, probably no more than twenty years old, his head shaved bald except for a barely raised Mohawk-stripe of nearly iridescent, nuclear green hair, rose from where he had been sitting cross-legged on the counter. Thin silver chains, hanging from his belt loops, made a tinkling sound as he shuffled to where his customers were pulling out chairs and seating themselves at a table.

Hartley was evidently a regular. "Just coffee," he said. "Any milk or cream for you, Doc?" A shake of Gottlieb's head sent the boy wordlessly behind the counter, where he began to fiddle with the coffee machine.

"Thanks again for taking a minute. I wasn't entirely truthful back there on the corner. There is something that's been bothering me. It's not about me, at least directly. It concerns a friend of mine named Tommy. Tommy Sawyer. I went back to New York last week when I got the word . . . you know, that he didn't have much longer."

Gottlieb nodded encouragingly. "You were worried about your friend. And now you're worried about yourself."

It was Hartley's turn to nod.

"How good a friend was he?"

Hartley looked around reflexively to see if somebody might be listening. Reassured that he and Gottlieb were the only customers in the place, he said emphatically, "Real good. It was two years ago. The summer of 1982. I got some time off and went back to New York. We spent the better part of a month together on Fire Island." Hartley paused for just a second.

"Tommy was different from my usual. I was mostly the one doing the social climbing. For him I was a step or two up the ladder. I honestly think that he's the first man I ever truly loved."

Gottlieb could tell this was the start of a much longer story. He had a patient whom he was supposed to see in clinic in a half hour. Nonetheless, he decided not to interrupt. He needed to find out where Hartley wanted to go with this. Kathy would take care of things until he could get back to the office. "So, what happened?" he asked.

"What I didn't know was that Tommy had a problem with drugs. It had been going on for a long time, but I swear he was clean when we went to the Island."

"How were things between the two of you once you got there?" Gottlieb asked.

"We were great. The sun was warm. The sand felt good between our toes. It was a place where the gay glitterati went, summer after summer. You could be uninhibited, as gay as you wanted to be. It was like a respite from the rest of the world, where, when we wanted, it was just the two of us and no one could intrude. Everything was low-key. Cars aren't allowed, so we hauled our stuff around in one of those little red wagons kids play with. You know, American Flyer."

Hartley emphasized that not all of Fire Island was gay. "There were two gay villages," he said. "One was called The Pines. That was where the rich people spent their summer. The Pines was about big houses and land-scaped yards. We rented a ramshackle cottage in Cherry Point. To get from The Pines to Cherry Point, you crossed a rustic stretch of forest everyone called the Meat Rack. The Meat Rack was especially popular after dark. There were plenty of secluded spots. We'd usually sleep till at least noon then go to somebody's house for cocktails, maybe spend some time on the beach. There'd be pre-parties every night at someone's house. Afterwards, we'd go dancing at Monster or another one of the clubs. We'd get back to the cottage around two or three, get some sleep, and start all over again the next day. Everyone was on drugs . . . cocaine just to keep going . . . ethyl chloride for sex . . . halcyon for sleep." Hartley's voice dropped lower.

"It sounds like you were really living it up. What happened to you and Tommy?" Gottlieb asked.

"Summer ended. We went back to the city, and I didn't hear from him. He didn't answer my calls. I was afraid that maybe he was sick, so I went downtown to where he'd told me he lived, down in the East Village. It took me a while but I finally found him. A real flophouse. He was completely zoned out. He smelled like he hadn't taken a bath in a week. In the past it had always been cocaine. He'd fallen in love with speedballs.[1] I couldn't compete. I'd had my own trouble with drugs, mostly coke and poppers. It had been bad enough that I didn't want to go back to where I'd been. I'm not proud of it, but I decided to save myself. I left Tommy lying there. It was the last time I'd seen him until I went to visit him in the hospital."

Gottlieb looked down at his cup. He was surprised to see that it was empty.

"More coffee, Doc?"

"I'm sorry, Brad, for you and for Tommy, but I've got a patient waiting for me at the clinic. I've got to get going."

"Sure, Doc. You've been terrific. Really, thanks for listening."

"I think you know that I should see you in the office for a checkup and a look at your T-cells," Gottlieb told him. "We can continue our conversation. I think I've got some time available next week. You'll call and make an appointment?"

"You can count on it, Doc. You head out and take care of things. I've got the tab."

Hartley stood and watched Gottlieb leave. He held up a finger and signaled the boy behind the counter for another cup of coffee. In his mind's eye, he could see Tommy as he was that summer on Fire Island, lean and darkly tanned. He had been a beautiful man. Now his face was ruined. Raised purple lumps strewn like hideous little islands on a graying lagoon. He'd lost a lot of weight. It had been difficult watching him. Worse than that, really. Hartley had to admit it: it had taken all of his strength to stay by Tommy's bedside.

He had left the hospital with every intention to return the next day. He'd promised Tommy as much. He cursed himself for his cowardice. The rest of the week he'd spent wandering the streets or drinking with friends, the ones who weren't sick yet. The ones he could still talk to. So many of his friends had died. Soon it would be Tommy's turn . . . if it hadn't happened already.

One of the evenings in New York, when he was at loose ends, he'd gone alone to the theater. Larry Kramer's *The Normal Heart* had recently opened off-Broadway at The Public Theater. Brad had never seen anything like it. It was as though he were a voyeur, witnessing vignettes from his own life, spoken in his own words. Kramer's protagonist, Ned Weeks, was afflicted with the same hostility toward the heterosexual world that Hartley felt. Like Weeks, he kept his emotions well concealed. He was a gay man living in limbo: neither fully part of society nor exempt from its rules and customs. In so many ways, Weeks spoke to Hartley's own growing resentment.

At its most basic level, Kramer's play was a cry for recognition of a gay America that was just beginning to emerge from its anonymity. Gay men were starting to face the intimidating prospect of announcing their homosexuality. Despite the backlash against authoritarian violence following the invasion of the Stonewall Inn, police and even common citizens continued to harass gay men on the slightest pretext. Twenty-nine states and the District of Columbia had laws on their books that forbade homosexual acts and prescribed criminal penalties. Until 1973 the American Psychiatric Association had considered homosexuality a mental disorder.

Despite the legal hangover, things were slowly changing. Fifteen years had passed since the Stonewall riots. What had been accomplished during that time, more than anything else, was a growing appreciation among members of the gay community that gay men had the right, as much as straight men, to exercise their personal freedom. Both symbolically and quite literally, that freedom was enacted nightly in acts of sexual abandonment. Sex, simply for the pleasure of it, without apologies and with no expectations of future responsibility, became a hallmark of the gay revolution.

Most unfortunately, AIDS appeared on the scene at the exact moment when gay sexual emancipation was becoming sufficiently visible that it achieved public recognition. Early medical publications concerning AIDS uniformly drew associations between homosexual promiscuity and the rising number of men dying from the newly discovered disease. Among straight Americans, the fear of AIDS changed the narrative of gay sexual liberation from ignorant curiosity to heightened hostility.

The Normal Heart captures the anger of gay men trying to make their way in straight society. Ned Weeks progressively becomes more confrontational as he faces the impossibility of achieving inclusion for those he represents and of convincing civic authorities to provide money to fight what straight society perceived to be a gay epidemic. As portrayed in the play, the silence surrounding AIDS spoke to an epidemic that no one wished to own up to, one in which suffering and death were tolerated specifically because they affected a minority group of individuals who already were treated as outcasts.

The complicity among members of a society that remains silent when their neighbors are dying all around them is a consistent theme of Kramer's writing. Despite self-evident differences between passive neglect and programmed genocide, Kramer frequently draws a controversial analogy between heterosexual America's ignoring the AIDS epidemic and the silence of ordinary German citizens during the Jewish Holocaust of World War II. Indeed, Kramer has said that it was while he was touring the concentration camp at Dachau that he conceived the idea for *The Normal Heart*.[2]

In Kramer's works, there is plenty of blame to go around. Kramer's unstinting characterization of homosexual promiscuity as the paramount factor in spreading AIDS earned him the scorn of some critics, who saw in his indictment of gay sexual adventurism nothing less than toadying to the mores of straight society and retrenchment from hard-won personal freedoms.

Despite the ruling gay dialectic, however, Kramer's position on promiscuity was consistent with the prevailing scientific view. Dr. Marcus Conant, the prominent, openly gay physician and AIDS researcher who had negotiated the Willie Brown grants to UCSF and UCLA, was an outspoken proponent of sexual restraint.[3] Conant argued that gay men are raised from childhood with the same social goals as heterosexuals. He asserted that gay men are taught the same ideal of a perfect and lasting union with a single individual. As they recognize their attraction to other men, however, and experience the urgency of sexual desire, they are torn by the dissonance between what they have been led to believe and the reality of gay sexual opportunity. They become conflicted between pressures to conform to the mores of straight society and the appeal of anonymous, impromptu sex proffered by the bathhouses and dance clubs that hosted the gay sexual revolution of the 1970s and 1980s.

According to Conant, despite all the evidence pointing to promiscuity as a risk factor for contracting AIDS, the emergence of the epidemic failed to change the sexual calculus. AIDS instilled fear among sexually active gay men but did not change their behavior. Why? Conant attributed much of the lethargic response to the emergence of AIDS to the human capacity for denial. In his experience, each man had his talisman, a rationalization by which he warded off confronting the possibility that he might be susceptible to developing AIDS.

As one example, Conant noted that even in the absence of epidemiological evidence, it was apparent to most that the disease was passed sexually. If this were the case, then by the simple laws of probability, the more partners with whom a man had sexual contact and the greater the frequency with which he indulged in sexual activity, the more likely he would be to develop AIDS. The problem Conant faced in convincing his patients that this was the case lay in the randomness of those same laws of probability. Conant related seeing in his office young men who would argue that because they had acquaintances who took on three or more sexual partners a day yet remained healthy, their own experiences of three partners per week or three per month or having a long-term relationship in which one or both partners occasionally indulged in sexual assignations outside the relationship couldn't be dangerous. Others argued that having sex on dirty sheets or having athlete's foot and walking barefoot on carpeting where others had recently had sex was the real culprit in passing the disease. Because of their intense attachment to a dangerous lifestyle, these men had managed to convince themselves of their invincibility—that by simply changing the sheets or wearing bath shoes they could avoid becoming another statistic of the epidemic.

Worst of all, Conant noted, was the coping mechanism he repeatedly observed among gay men when an acquaintance came down with AIDS. Although never spoken aloud, "out of sight, out of mind" was the prevailing mantra. So long as a man did not actually have to see the afflicted individual or speak with him, he could convince himself that, despite their similar sexual proclivities, he was not at risk.

As illustrated by *The Normal Heart*, how gay men denied the evident risk during the early years of the epidemic makes sense in the context of the times. Many gay men were forced to lead two lives: by day they were productive, well-integrated members of a heterosexual work environment, haunted by the fear that exposure of their sexual predilections might mean termination of their employment, or even prosecution; by night, the same men exorcised their daytime fears by living out their sexual compulsion. The expression of hypersexuality was such a feature of gay life, such a symbol of emancipation from heterosexual strictures, that even well-respected voices like Kramer's and Conant's thought more than once before giving vent to their concerns. No one wished to be accused of being against sex, the self-hating one who put an end to the good times.

Hartley's week in New York had been an emotionally exhausting one. He considered ordering one more cup of coffee. *One more and you'll have even more trouble than usual getting to sleep*, he thought and decided against it. He made a mental note to call for an appointment and get that checkup Gottlieb had recommended. Really though, why should he? *I'm feeling fine*, he thought. *I know a lot of guys who are having more sex than me, and they're doing fine, too. Actually, not so many . . . but a few. They haven't caught the disease.* He would get around to seeing Gottlieb when things slowed down.

EIGHT

Rock

Michael Gottlieb's office assistant put through a telephone call one afternoon in early June 1984. What he and the caller discussed would lead to his caring for the first major celebrity to acknowledge having and eventually dying of AIDS. In time, the episode would link Gottlieb to the entertainment community and raise questions in the minds of his superiors about his seriousness as an academic physician.

The caller was Dr. Letantia Bussell, a dermatologist whose Beverly Hills practice reputedly included many of LA's well-known and wealthy. Despite her never having met Gottlieb, she advised him that she wished to speak with him in confidence and that the need for discretion was paramount. Intrigued, he promised confidentiality and asked her to continue.

Dr. Bussell had recently biopsied a purplish nodule on the arm of one of her patients, the film star Rock Hudson. An apocryphal story has it that Hudson had first been made aware of the small skin growth by Nancy Reagan, who was said to have noticed it during a Hudson visit to the White House. The pathologist's report had returned a diagnosis of Kaposi's sarcoma. Bussell suspected that Hudson had AIDS. To minimize the possibility that the media would catch wind of things, she asked Gottlieb if he would be willing to assess Hudson in her office.

Bussell and Gottlieb decided on June 5, 1984, as the date Gottlieb would examine Hudson. Coincidentally, it was exactly three years to the day after the publication in *Morbidity and Mortality Weekly Report* of Gottlieb's article describing a new syndrome of decreased cellular immunity and atypical pneumonia in five gay men. "I got into my 1977 Dodge Aspen station wagon and drove over there," he said. "I don't think I'd ever even been to Beverly Hills before."[1]

Gottlieb was met by an office assistant, who admitted him to a large, well-decorated space that appeared to be a combined office and examination room. Dr. Bussell greeted him and introduced him to Rock Hudson as the doctor with the greatest experience in caring for people with findings like his. Gottlieb also shook hands with Hudson's personal physician, Dr. Rex Kenemer, whose practice reputedly included as patients a number of film industry celebrities. Kenemer acknowledged that he had little experience in dealing with AIDS. He expressed the wish that if the diagnosis of AIDS were confirmed, Gottlieb would take over that aspect of Hudson's care. When Gottlieb agreed, Bussell and Kenemer exited, leaving him alone with Rock Hudson.

Hudson and Gottlieb sat across from each other and spoke for about thirty minutes. The conversation was personable and directed toward Hudson's health concerns. Gottlieb's first impression of Hudson was that he was a kindly, quiet sort of man who might be used to letting things take their natural course. Gottlieb later learned that Hudson's homosexuality was well known in Hollywood and the California gay community, but at this first meeting, neither of the men addressed Hudson's sexual preferences, nor did they discuss how he might have contracted the disease. Indeed, Gottlieb said he made it a point not to ask how his patients acquired HIV for fear of their feeling embarrassed and becoming alienated early in the course of establishing their relationship.

Gottlieb asked Hudson to sit on the edge of Bussell's examination table so that he could take a look at him. What he noticed first was that Hudson was a big man, six feet four inches tall. "I had to look upward in order to make eye contact, and that surprised me, as I was six feet tall, myself," Gottlieb recalled. Hudson seemed thin for his height but not in the haggard, wasted way that AIDS patients can look when they reach the end-stage of their disease. He acknowledged that he recently had lost some weight. Otherwise, Gottlieb's physical examination turned up nothing remarkable beyond his having several other small, nodular Kaposi's lesions like the one on his arm.

Dr. Gottlieb told Hudson that he believed he had AIDS, and that there was no treatment, but researchers were working on something. The diagnosis confirmed what Hudson had feared. He told Gottlieb that he had written anonymous letters to several recent sexual contacts warning them that they had been exposed to someone carrying the virus. He'd had the letters sent without his signature from a postal address outside the Los Angeles area. Gottlieb inferred that he intended the precautions to minimize the possibility of his being blackmailed.

Hudson asked Gottlieb whether that was what he thought he should have done. Gottlieb was unsure whether the question was rhetorical or Hudson really wanted an answer. He replied with a question of his own, "Is that what you wanted to do?"

"I wanted to do the right thing," Hudson responded.

"I drew some blood to look at his T-cells and labeled the tube Roy Harold Scherer Jr., the name Hudson told me his parents had given him at his birth," Gottlieb said. He returned to his office and handed the tube to his lab assistant, Kathryn Petersilie.

Petersilie was not fooled by Gottlieb's crude attempt at providing his patient with anonymity. She recalled, "I looked at the tube, and I said this is Rock Hudson."[2]

"How do you know?" Gottlieb asked.

"Because I'm a big fan. You have to use another name," she urged.

Petersilie was not alone in her devotion to the popular actor. Hudson was born in Winnetka, Illinois, on November 17, 1925. His mother was a telephone operator, his father an auto mechanic who abandoned the family during the Depression. Still a young boy, he became Roy Fitzgerald when his mother remarried and his stepfather adopted him.

Those who knew him when he was growing up remember Hudson as being unusually shy. As a teenager he earned spending money doing odd jobs, delivering newspapers, and caddying at the local golf course. An undistinguished student, he graduated from New Trier High School, then joined the military and served in the Pacific during World War II. At the end of hostilities, he landed in Los Angeles, thinking he'd give acting a try.

At first he scrounged for whatever acting jobs he could find while doing odd jobs and driving a truck to keep fed and housed. The University of Southern California rejected Hudson's application to its film school. Eventually, however, he managed to attract the attention of talent scout Harry

Willson, who became his agent. It was Willson who dubbed the young Roy Fitzgerald "Rock Hudson," a name Hudson hated but stuck with for the rest of his life.

Under Willson's tutelage, Hudson soon snagged his first leading role, playing opposite Jean Wyman in the acclaimed 1954 film *Magnificent Obsession*. His performance made him an international star. Fans voted Hudson the year's most popular actor, and his career took off. His several romantic roles opposite Doris Day, of which *Pillow Talk* is the best known, and his versatility in making a total of seventy films covering nearly every imaginable genre, made him one of the most sought after leading men of his generation.

As his film career began to fade during the early 1970s, Hudson, seemingly effortlessly, turned to television. He had a successful seven-year run with Susan St. James in the highly rated detective series *McMillan and Wife*. At the time Gottlieb diagnosed him as having AIDS, Hudson was playing Linda Evans's love interest on the prime-time soap opera *Dynasty*. It was only as he weakened and began to have difficulty delivering his lines that the writers killed off his character, simultaneously terminating both the fictitious Daniel Reece and Rock Hudson's prodigious acting career.

From their first meeting, Gottlieb honored Hudson's caution over the public learning about his condition. Hudson never came to Gottlieb's clinic or office at UCLA, for fear of exposure by the snitches the media were said to have planted among the medical center employees or the entertainment beat reporters and paparazzi who frequented the entrances to the medical center on the off chance that some celebrity might be caught unaware. While some film stars might sneak by in disguise, it would be hard to conceal the identity of a man whose physique and reputation loomed as large as Rock Hudson's.

When there was a need to meet, Gottlieb would arrange to see Hudson either at Dr. Bussell's office or at Hudson's rambling, Spanish-style home in the canyons above Beverly Hills. Known as "The Castle," Hudson's house was perched on a hillside and had several terraces to take in the surrounding views. The residence was also home to one of Hudson's former lovers, Tom Clark, and his personal assistant, Mark Miller. Hudson's accountant and business manager Wally Sheft and his publicist Dale Olson were frequent visitors.

Hudson's home was his refuge, where he could meet Gottlieb and feel that his privacy was secure. It also was the place where he received his lovers while maintaining the self-deception that his sexual preference remained a secret. One Hudson paramour, Lee Garlington, told of how he would awaken early in the morning, leave by 6:30, and soundlessly coast his car down the hill toward town before he started the engine so the neighbors wouldn't notice his departure. According to Garlington, these kinds of precautions weren't paranoid behavior. The actor was just being realistic. It was "career suicide," Garlington said, to come out during that era. Hudson took extra steps to secure his property after a woman stalker gained access to The Castle one weekend when he was out of town, building a high fence and adding locked gates as impediments to the entry of uninvited guests.[3]

At the time Hudson presented with AIDS, Gottlieb was in frequent contact with Jean-Claude Chermann, one of his friends at the Pasteur Institute. Chermann had made him aware of a new therapeutic agent, HPA-23, being tested in Paris under the supervision of a French naval physician, Dr. Dominique Dormont. The intravenously administered drug had shown some value in fighting retroviral infections in animals and was then in early-phase clinical trials in human subjects, including a small number of Americans who had grown desperate enough to travel in search of a viable treatment. Gottlieb suggested Hudson go to Paris to give it a try and made arrangements for his introduction to Dr. Dormont.

Shortly before the 1985 Cannes Film Festival, which Hudson was scheduled to attend, Gottlieb received a call from Mark Miller. His boss wasn't feeling well. Two days earlier, Hudson had made an unfortunate appearance on the television show *Doris Day's Best Friends*. He was haggard looking and nearly incomprehensible when he spoke, and the appearance shocked many of his fans.[4] Miller wanted to know whether Hudson should make the trip or cancel his plans for Cannes. There was no time for Gottlieb to examine Hudson. Miller's responses to Gottlieb's questions concerning Hudson's condition failed to elicit any sign that his patient might be about to crash. Gottlieb advised Miller that ultimately the decision should depend on how Hudson felt, but that he saw no reason why he couldn't proceed with his plans. Gottlieb also suggested that if there were time, Hudson should make a stop in Paris for an infusion of HPA-23.

Hudson's decision to travel to France turned out to be a mistake. On July 21, while awaiting HPA-23 treatment in the Ritz Hotel, Hudson collapsed in the lobby. He was rushed to the American Hospital of Paris, where a CT scan of his abdomen revealed that he had developed a tumor in his liver. A biopsy confirmed the diagnosis of non-Hodgkin's lymphoma, a cancer commonly associated with AIDS.

Mark Miller, who was traveling with Hudson, contacted the Parisian publicist Yanou Collart, a friend of Hudson's, and told her that his boss had AIDS.[5] Initially, Collart publicly denied that Hudson had the disease, attributing the fainting episode to the liver tumor. However, two days later, after the actor had undergone extensive testing, Collart reversed herself, saying that Hudson did in fact have AIDS. She claimed that Hudson had contracted the disease from a blood transfusion given him a few years earlier during a quintuple coronary artery bypass procedure. In fact, since the episode occurred prior to the development of an accurate test for AIDS, tainted blood administered during surgery may well have been the actual cause of Hudson's AIDS.[6] Regardless, the aroused French media indulged themselves in lurid speculation.

A series of administrative problems plagued Hudson's hospitalization. First, as Dormont was a military doctor, he had no license to treat a patient in a civil hospital. It was only after waiting for a personal petition from President Reagan to French president Francois Mitterand that never came that Dormont received permission from the Ministry of the French Army to proceed with infusing the HPA-23.[7]

The public interest in Hudson's condition and the media response thoroughly disrupted the French hospital's operations. After about a week the hospital informed Hudson's retinue that it would prefer that Hudson be treated in the United States.[8] Soon thereafter, Gottlieb received a telephone call from Pierre Salinger. At that time, the former Kennedy and Johnson administrations' press secretary was working in London as the ABC television network's chief foreign correspondent. Salinger told Gottlieb that Collart had called and asked him to help facilitate Hudson's return to the United States. "He wants to come back to Los Angeles to be with people he knows,"[9] Salinger said. Gottlieb agreed to receive Hudson in transfer and admit him to UCLA.

To get Hudson home, Salinger chartered an Air France B-747 at a cost of $250,000. He had the seats in the first class section removed and a hospital bed bolted to the floor. The flight left Paris late in the afternoon of July 30, with Rock Hudson and his medical attendants as its sole passengers. The plane arrived at Los Angeles International Airport around 11 o'clock that evening. Hudson was transferred by stretcher from the airplane to a helicopter waiting to take him across town on the last leg of his journey to UCLA.

By 1984, in part due to Gottlieb's work, the fortunes of the CIA had improved both literally and metaphorically. The institution had swapped out the CIA's basement labs and offices for larger, airier, more prestigious digs on the fifth floor. Past midnight, Gottlieb walked from his office to the south side of the hospital, overlooking the emergency helipad, and watched the helicopter ferrying Hudson from LAX to the medical center parry with several circling news choppers for airspace over the hospital helipad. This was the story the news media had come to witness and recount: a famous man, who had been diagnosed with AIDS, arriving by helicopter. Hang the risk; the public would not be denied its due.

Gottlieb met Hudson in the emergency room, then waited while the stricken actor was admitted to a private room on the tenth floor of the hospital, the limited access floor reserved for the moneyed and famous. He waited a while longer for the intern, David Aboulafia, to complete his medical history and physical examination. UCLA was a teaching hospital. Every patient was a potential teaching case. Admitting procedures would not be abrogated, even for an in extremis movie star.

When Gottlieb finally saw Hudson, it was nearly 3:00 a.m. Hudson was feverish and short of breath. His chest X-ray showed signs of pneumonia. Gottlieb assumed that his patient had a *Pneumocystis* infection of his lungs. "Rock was pretty much out of it," Gottlieb said. "He was not comatose, but not really very responsive to questions, either." He placed Hudson on antibiotic treatment appropriate for *Pneumocystis* pneumonia, and his patient responded over the next several days. "He got somewhat better, but never really did great," said Gottlieb.

Inevitably, Gottlieb became embroiled in the media glare that surrounds celebrities. "When Rock Hudson became my patient and the eyes of the world were focused on the UCLA Medical Center, and Rock Hudson became the face that people recognized as being the face of AIDS, it got much worse," he remembered. "My being Rock Hudson's physician certainly attracted a lot of national attention."

"I believe that there were UCLA faculty who were proud of my involvement and of the attention it brought to the plight of patients with AIDS," he noted. However, Gottlieb sensed irritation on the part of the hospital administration that UCLA was being so openly associated with AIDS. He also had another problem: several prominent members of the faculty wanted to take part in Hudson's care. It was at times like these that Gottlieb felt the most insecure. He was a thirty-five-year-old, untenured assistant professor. Lacking the advice of a trusted mentor, he was flying alone across uncharted territory. He sorely felt the pressures that could be exerted by the icons of the institution.

"There [were] people on the faculty who demanded to see the patient, demanded to be called in to consult, and when I said 'no,' [they] got angry. I should have been much more political and said 'Oh, of course.'"

The chair of the Department of Psychiatry, Dr. Louis Jolyon West, known as "Jolly" and renowned for his work with LSD, phoned to offer his services. Gottlieb declined. "I didn't think [Hudson] needed a psychiatric consult. I don't know where [West] was coming from."

Reminiscent of his call to Marcus Conant promising to scuttle the legislative grant that Willie Brown had brokered if his demands weren't met, David Golde told Gottlieb in what the latter perceived to be a threatening tone, "I want to be involved." Gottlieb also declined this request. "He was always after the money, and that caused me to view him with some suspicion," Gottlieb said of Golde. "That caused some hard feelings."

The relationship between Gottlieb and Golde took another step backward when Gottlieb sought a consultant from Golde's Division of Oncology to work up the tumor in Hudson's liver that the French physicians had discovered in Paris. Without discussing it with Golde, he asked that the lymphoma specialist, Dr. Greg Sarna, see his patient to confirm the diagnosis and determine what, if any, treatment might be appropriate.

Gottlieb knew at the time that choosing Sarna might cause him trouble. Ronald Mitsuyasu, a developing young clinician researcher, was Golde's favorite. Golde had assigned Mitsuyasu to take over the Kaposi's sarcoma clinic after Jerome Groopman's departure. Failing to ask him to participate in the Hudson case posed some risk. So Gottlieb was disappointed but not surprised when he heard that his choice had offended both Golde and Mitsuyasu. Gottlieb said that he'd made the decision based solely on what he felt was best for his patient. He ticked off the considerations that had led to his decision: Sarna was an experienced faculty oncologist who'd subspecialized in the care of lymphoma patients and had a broad range of experience. Mitsuyasu was still in fellowship training and lacked Sarna's breadth of experience and lymphoma-specific expertise.

The episode earned Gottlieb a few new enemies and even drew a negative comment from his department chair. In acknowledging that he had spent much more time dealing with issues related to Gottlieb than an assistant professor usually warranted, Shine said, "He was pleasant, almost charming, with a knowledge of the issues, but in my opinion, he needed to change his behavior and he did not change his behavior a whit. That was especially true of his relationships with his colleagues. I believe he could have changed those relationships early on if he'd chosen to, but he chose not to."[10]

From the moment Hudson was admitted, the press clamored for news. Was it true that the actor had AIDS? How had he caught it? What was his condition? Was he gay? The last of these questions was the one both Hudson and Gottlieb wished to avoid, so at first Gottlieb issued no response. Instead, he visited Hudson daily, sitting for a time on the edge of Hudson's hospital bed, neither he nor his patient saying much of consequence.

Finally, after almost a week following the admission, the medical center's public relations director, John Pontarelli, approached Gottlieb: "They're driving us crazy," he said, speaking of the news media. "We've got to say something." Gottlieb asked Hudson if it was alright for him to confirm for the media his diagnosis of AIDS. Hudson responded, "Go ahead and tell them if you think it will do any good."

The press conference was held at midday in the yawning UCLA Neuropsychiatric Institute auditorium. Gottlieb decided that, as Hudson's physician, he should make the announcement. "I realized it was a big moment in the history of the epidemic, and I wanted it. . . . I grabbed the spotlight," he said, acknowledging that this at least was one time when Shine's charge that he was "publicity seeking" might have had some validity. The administration acquiesced. On Pontarelli's advice, Gottlieb would read a brief, prepared statement confirming that his patient had AIDS and was being treated for AIDS-related complications at UCLA Medical Center. Neither Gottlieb nor anyone else was to answer reporters' questions.

"I was so hamstrung by the institution that I simply read a statement and declined to answer questions, much to the frustration of the gathered press." In the end, Gottlieb regretted that he had told them no more than what they already knew.

Responding to the hospitalization, Hudson improved to the point that he was well enough for Gottlieb to consider the eventual disposition of his patient. Greg Sarna's consultation didn't pull any punches: Hudson's liver tumor was inoperable and unlikely to be responsive to chemotherapy. Sarna's conclusions made official what Gottlieb had known for some time: Hudson was dying. He made preparations to send his patient home with measures to assure his comfort, ultimately discharging him from the hospital in late August 1985.

This outcome suited all concerned. Hudson would live out what remained of his life in familiar surroundings, in the company of his friends. The media frenzy that had been disrupting hospital operations would abandon the medical center for something fresher in the news cycle. UCLA's institutional administrators would put aside their fears of excessive public attention too closely linking their hospital to AIDS, which they feared was negatively affecting their institutional image. And the medical center's physicians and staff could return their full attention to the business of providing health care.

Once he returned home, Hudson continued to receive visits from friends and use what time he had left to make more visible to the public the ravages of the AIDS epidemic. In September he sent a telegram to the organizers of a Los Angeles AIDS benefit, Commitment to Life, which he had been invited to but was too sick to attend. Burt Lancaster read Hudson's statement to the crowd: "I am not happy that I am sick. I am not happy that I have AIDS. But if that is helping others, I can at least know that my own misfortune has had some positive worth."[11]

Prominent members of the Hollywood community applauded his openness and courage. Actress Morgan Fairchild opined that by revealing his condition, Hudson had put a face on the deadly disease.[12] Comedian Joan Rivers said, "Rock's admission is a horrendous way to bring AIDS to the attention of the American public, but by doing so, Rock, in his life, has helped millions in the process. What Rock has done takes true courage."[13]

Inevitably there were those who questioned the authenticity of Hudson's message. Film producer Ross Hunter, who had hired Hudson for a number of his films and claimed to be his closest friend, said that Hudson had been unaware of the worldwide interest in his disease and had not been cognizant of the message read at the gala. Hunter based his doubts on his perception during his visits to the actor's home that Hudson was lucid for only a few minutes at a time.[14] "Had Rock been well enough to be aware of the banquet and all the publicity," he said, "I'm sure he would have hated it. He was a very private person and never liked to discuss his personal life or problems with anyone."

The next day Hunter backpedaled on a number of his assertions, saying that he had not wished to cast doubts upon the veracity of Dale Olson. The publicist said that he had worked directly with his client in crafting the message and received Hudson's approval for it to be read at the Commitment to Life event. Hudson's lawyer, Paul Sherman, confirmed that his client had been lucid and given his assent.

Hudson died at his home on the morning of October 2, 1985. He was cremated the same day and his ashes scattered on the Pacific Ocean. The actor left instructions that there should be neither a wake nor a memorial service. Nonetheless, Gottlieb joined Hudson's many friends in commemorating his death with a celebration of his life. Guests filled the rooms of The Castle and overflowed onto the terraces, where a catering service served margaritas. Mariachis meandered among the crowd, singing loudly and playing their instruments.

Despite the fact that Hudson's friends knew that he was dying, the reactions to his death expressed surprise and compassion. President Ronald Reagan issued a White House press release that skirted the thorny issue of how his friend had died by writing: "Nancy and I are saddened by the news of Rock Hudson's death. He will always be remembered for his dynamic impact on the film industry, and fans all over the world will certainly mourn his loss. He will be remembered for his humanity, his sympathetic spirit, and well-deserved reputation for kindness. May God rest his soul."[15]

Elizabeth Taylor, who had been a frequent visitor to The Castle, commented that her time with Hudson had brought her closer to her friend in his final days. She issued a short statement: "I love him and tragically he is gone. Please God, he did not die in vain." Taylor asked that in lieu of flowers, friends of Hudson should consider a contribution to the newly announced American Foundation for AIDS Research (amfAR), for which she was the national spokeswoman.[16]

In how he comported himself during his prolonged and very public illness and in his death, Hudson gave visibility to a disease that, because of its association with homosexuality, many had wished to sweep from public view. Actress Linda Evans encapsulated this sentiment: "As fine an actor as Rock was, and as much as he shared his craft with us, I feel that his greatest gift to the world was in his acknowledgment of his disease and in his willingness to educate people and raise their consciousness."[17]

The public reaction was overwhelmingly sympathetic, and several days after Hudson's death, Congress set aside $221 million to conduct research on finding a cure for AIDS. One prominent AIDS advocate, Bruce Decker, commented at the time, "Hudson's illness and death have moved the fight against AIDS ahead more in three months than anything in the previous three years."[18]

In America's executive branch of government, however, perceptions of AIDS changed more slowly. Most of Reagan's appointees viewed AIDS indifferently or with antagonism. Surgeon General C. Everett Koop was the exception. In 1986 Koop convinced the president to allow him to draft a report on AIDS. Later that year he released it to the press without first allowing the report to be vetted by Reagan's domestic advisers.[19] A year later, in 1987, he released a condensed version to every household in America recommending that all public schools provide AIDS education.

On May 31, 1987, about the time Koop's report was reaching mailboxes and near the end of Ronald Reagan's second term, selected physicians and researchers attending the Third International Conference on AIDS in Washington, D.C., boarded a bus and were taken to a restaurant in Georgetown, along the waterfront. Michael and Cindy Gottlieb were among them. Following lunch, the crowd was ushered into a tent erected earlier that day to house the president's first address on the AIDS epidemic. Cindy Gottlieb recalls being shown to a reserved seat in the second row. Nancy and Ronald Reagan entered the tent to the strains of "Hail to the Chief," and Mrs. Reagan took her seat next to Elizabeth Taylor, immediately in front of Cindy. Her husband sat alongside Ms. Taylor.

As the crowd settled itself, the evening's master of ceremonies introduced Elizabeth Taylor. Gottlieb rose to escort her to the podium. After brief introductory remarks, she made a presentation honoring Surgeon General Koop for his courage and persistence in making the AIDS epidemic a national priority. Two more recognitions followed. Gottlieb presented an award to Dr. Robert Gallo for his groundbreaking work with retroviruses. The New York socialite and AIDS activist Mathilde Krim presented a similar appreciation to the Pasteur Institute's Dr. Luc Montagnier.[20]

The president's speech, during which he finally addressed the AIDS epidemic, was no less historic for its brevity. At one point Reagan mentioned potentially requiring mandatory testing as a policy to combat AIDS. This was anathema to many in the crowd, who viewed mandatory testing as homophobic and an abrogation of civil rights, and some of the attendees began to boo and heckle Reagan. Elizabeth Taylor rose to his defense, shouting, "Don't be rude. This is your President and he is our guest."[21]

Policy differences aside, for the first time AIDS received presidential recognition. President Reagan had publicly acknowledged the existence of a disease that during the previous six years had claimed the lives of more than twenty thousand Americans and spread to 113 countries around the world.[22] Reagan's speech was not simply the end of an era of ostrich-like government avoidance of a national crisis. It was the beginning of societal recognition that the epidemic had progressed from being nearly exclusively a disease of gay men to one that threatened men and women, straight and gay, adults and children.

That evening in 1987, alongside Washington's Potomac River, when President Reagan first addressed the AIDS epidemic, was bittersweet for Gottlieb. He undoubtedly weighed the satisfaction of hearing long-sought presidential recognition of AIDS against the emotional toll he'd paid during his years-long battle with UCLA and its institutional leadership. Looking back on the hectic months during which he had cared for Rock Hudson, Gottlieb said that the episode dramatically and negatively impacted his career at UCLA. His dedication to Hudson and all that went along with caring for the actor had sufficiently interfered with his normal activities that he had fallen behind in his commitments. He made this explicit in an August 20, 1985, letter responding to senior immunologist John Fahey's concerns about delays in Gottlieb's promised support in helping write a planned federal grant application: "Thank you for your note. I hope you understand that caring for Rock Hudson has been a full-time job. I am hopeful that our part in providing his medical care will enhance our immunology and AIDS programs at UCLA. As you know, I am coordinating anti-virals and immunotherapy trials for HTLV-III infection complicated by infections and lymphadenopathy at UCLA. I would like to discuss these as they relate to the above RFA [request for applications[23]] at your earliest convenience."[24]

Gottlieb said, "Here I was in this tiny division with only a part-time secretary. It should have been obvious to even a casual observer that the stresses related to taking care of Rock Hudson, in addition to all of my usual responsibilities, were overwhelming. No one from my department or the administration reached out to offer any support."

Ken Shine confirmed that the Hudson episode had negatively colored how he and, he believed, other faculty viewed Gottlieb. In amplification,

Shine cited an episode that he said occurred during Hudson's hospitalization that summed up his concerns about Gottlieb's priorities:

> One day I'm in the corridor and Rock Hudson had been admitted. I met him [Gottlieb] in the hallway, and he had a whole bunch of pink telephone slips. And I said, "What's that all about." And he said, "It's about fifty-five calls that I've got to return." I said, "What do you mean by fifty-five calls." And he said, "Well, I have all these people who want to know about Rock Hudson." So I said, "Does Mr. Hudson want you talking about him?" And he said, "Yes, he doesn't have any objection at all." So I said, "Why don't you hold a news conference instead of answering fifty-five phone calls." And he said, "Because there are a lot of influential people here, and I'm going to be able to make a lot of important connections that are very valuable."[25] So I found that he was spending huge amounts of time outside of his teaching and research activities in developing a social network.

Gottlieb remembered the conversation and felt that his former chairman's characterization had unfairly represented his motives. "Yes, I was cultivating connections to help the AIDS cause and with the goal of helping AIDS programs at the university get ahead," he said. He believed Shine had largely ignored the epidemic into which Gottlieb had thrown his every professional effort. "In retrospect, it should have been clear to me that their agenda was to deemphasize AIDS, and that was hard to do with Rock Hudson in the hospital. If he thought responding to phone calls was about star-fucking,[26] he was wrong. It wasn't."

Gottlieb believed that the Rock Hudson affair was lethal to his academic prospects: "There was a great deal of envy and jealousy about my being Rock's physician and a great deal of irritation on the part of the administration that UCLA had been so openly associated with being an AIDS center." His superiors' perceptions of Gottlieb's role in the Rock Hudson affair would haunt him throughout the remainder of his employment at the university. The episode had moved Michael Gottlieb from the eye of the storm to ground zero.

NINE

Elizabeth

Viewed as medical metaphor, the impact of the Rock Hudson affair on Gottlieb's relationships with his superiors had been an acute inflammatory event. Like a case of pneumonia, it was intense and over quickly but left a lasting scar to memorialize the hurt. Gottlieb's friendship with Elizabeth Taylor and his partnering with her on behalf of AIDS were something quite different—a chronic, festering irritant to his detractors that proved in their minds what they had thought about Gottlieb since his discovery of AIDS. He lacked the seriousness and focus required of an academic physician.

A legend developed around Gottlieb—part mythology, part reality— concerning his involvement with Hollywood celebrity in general and Elizabeth Taylor in particular. Andrew Saxon told a story that, though he was uncertain whether it was true, encapsulated why he had been concerned about Gottlieb's suitability for academic medicine: "I have this recall, and you better check it with Mike, that he canceled his promotion discussion with the Dean or with his chairman to have lunch with Elizabeth Taylor. And that's probably not true, but it's the anecdote I remember. He got suckered in by the glitz."[1]

Neither Gottlieb nor Ken Shine recalled anything of the kind having occurred. However, that Saxon remembered the story more than thirty years after its supposed occurrence and mentioned it a second time without the disclaimer in a later conversation raised the probability that he and others may have given credence to the rumor at the time.

Gottlieb first met Elizabeth Taylor in August 1985. She had come to the medical center to visit her friend, Rock Hudson, following his return to the United States from France. On that occasion, Taylor was accompanied by her personal assistant, Roger Wall; her publicist of twenty years, Chen Sam; and AIDS Project Los Angeles executive director Bill Misenhimer.

Gottlieb reported that he felt nervous at first, awed by Taylor's glamour and fame, but the film star quickly put him at ease. "It was her personality that was always larger-than-life," he said. "She had a lively sense of humor, a naturally hearty laugh, even though her visiting Hudson was a serious occasion. She was very down to earth."[2] Gottlieb especially appreciated Taylor's efforts to make him feel more comfortable. She told him, "I'm just a Jewish girl from Pasadena."[3]

Shortly after she met Gottlieb, Taylor phoned him directly to ask if he would do her a favor. On her first visit, she had found the media attention surrounding Hudson intimidating. She wanted to visit her friend again, but this time she wanted to escape the prying eyes of television news cameras and avoid the gauntlet of intrusively questioning reporters camped out in front of the medical center. She asked if there were some way she could see Hudson without attracting any attention. Gottlieb agreed to help.

The following Sunday morning, Gottlieb picked up Taylor at her Bel Air home and ferried her to a little used entrance at the rear of the hospital. From there he led the actress through a maze of windowless corridors to a marred, graffiti-streaked service elevator. Gottlieb pushed the call button and heard the machinery groan into action. When the elevator door opened, he selected the button for the tenth floor, setting into motion the elevator's slow ascent. Stealing a glance at his impeccably dressed, perfectly coiffed companion, Gottlieb recalled thinking how incongruously out of place Taylor looked in the dingy, haltingly functioning elevator.

The elevator stopped abruptly on the tenth floor. Precariously cantilevered on her stylish pumps, Taylor stumbled for an instant and almost fell. As she steadied herself, Gottlieb heard the loud clunk of something hard striking the elevator wall.

"What was that?" he asked.

Unruffled and laughing, Taylor held out her right hand and replied, "Oh. Just my jewels." In regaining her balance, she had inadvertently banged against the elevator's metal wall the thirty-two-carat Krupp diamond ring given her by Richard Burton.

Gottlieb led Taylor down a hallway and stopped outside of Hudson's room to update her on his medical status and give her some insight into what she could expect. On Taylor's first visit to see Hudson, he had been so ill that he was barely cognizant of her presence. Since then, he had greatly improved.

Seeming to Gottlieb to be a bit anxious, Taylor asked the young physician a number of questions. How close could she safely get to Hudson? Given Hudson's immune deficiency, what was the risk to him of her touching him? For how long could she stay? Once Gottlieb reassured her that normal contact would not put either of them in jeopardy, Taylor entered the room with brio. She hugged Hudson and kissed him on the cheek before sitting on the edge of his bed. Gottlieb left them alone for about an hour. He then secreted Taylor out of the building the way they had come in and returned her to Bel Air. "We bonded," Gottlieb said.

In her fifty-third year, Elizabeth Taylor was living a remarkable life. She was the second of two children born to American expatriates living in England. Her father, Francis, was a successful art dealer, while her mother, Sara, had been an actress before their marriage. The Taylors felt at home on the outskirts of London and had successfully ingratiated themselves with the British gentry. However, as World War II threatened to engulf Europe, the Taylors reluctantly returned to the United States.

They settled in Los Angeles, where the film industry got its first look at their daughter, Elizabeth. Even at age seven, Elizabeth was such a remarkable looking child that film studios vied to place her under contract. Her blue eyes—so dark that they appeared violet—paired with a genetic variation that graced her with a double layer of eyelashes, imparted a look that some felt was too frankly sexual for a child actress. Indeed, some of the photographs of the young Elizabeth depict her boldly staring at the viewer with an unafraid worldliness well beyond her years.

Taylor played her first major film role opposite Roddy McDowell in the 1943 film *Lassie Come Home*. A year later she won the iconic part of Velvet Brown, a young horsewoman obsessed with winning a national championship, in the huge hit *National Velvet*. The film paved Elizabeth's way to international stardom. However, even as studios clamored for her services, Taylor was proving she had a mind of her own. She bridled under the strict supervision of her mother and the studio educational program, which cut her off from contact with other children. She said, "As I got more famous—after *National Velvet,* when I was 12—I still wanted to be part of their (other children's) lives, but I think, in a way, they began to regard me as a sort of an oddity, a freak."[4]

As she transitioned to adult roles, Taylor's career blossomed. She won Academy Awards for Best Actress for *Butterfield 8* and *Who's Afraid of Virginia Woolf.* In the latter film, Taylor played the boozy, outrageously shrewish daughter of the president of a small college, married to a milque-toast faculty member, portrayed by her real-life husband, Richard Burton. She said of Burton, whom she married twice, that he was one of the three great loves of her life, the other two being her third husband, Michael Todd, and jewelry.[5] Wed eight times in all, Taylor led a tumultuous personal life. She had lifelong back and neck problems, which she attributed to a fall from horseback while filming *National Velvet.* As she aged, the back pain led her to a dependence on prescription pain medications.

Taylor knew Rock Hudson from their years working in the small Hollywood film community. They had grown close when they costarred in *Giant,* the only film for which Hudson received an Oscar nomination. One evening after filming for the day was complete, Hudson and Taylor got roaring drunk. Hudson said that they connected that night. It was when they had first really gotten to know each other, the start of their friendship.[6] Reminiscing about their times together after Hudson became symptomatic with AIDS, Taylor said, "Oh, God, yes, I knew he was gay, but I thought he had cancer."[7]

By the time Gottlieb met her in 1985, Taylor's career in films was all but over. Like Hudson, she had made forays into television, but her real interests lay elsewhere. Early that year she had received a visit from seven gay men she knew, who beseeched her to help them break the silence they felt surrounded AIDS in the film community.[8] At about the same time, her daughter-in-law and mother of her grandchildren, Aileen Getty, contracted HIV. Elizabeth Taylor foresaw a part for herself in improving the plight of people with AIDS. She anticipated the possibility of engaging in a cause much bigger than her next film role. Nonetheless, just as she had shrewdly waited for just the right part to play in a movie, she waited for an opportunity that was appropriate for her talents.

The chance to insert herself into the fight against AIDS soon appeared in the person of Bill Misenhimer. Early in the 1980s the openly gay Misenhimer was working in finance as an executive for Xerox. Through a special program offered by his employer, he successfully applied for a year's paid sabbatical to work for a small, homegrown, not-for-profit organization called AIDS Project Los Angeles (APLA). His friends were dying of AIDS, and he wished to join the fight against the deadly disease.

In 1984 APLA was a struggling, community-based nonprofit that helped its clients cope with their daily needs. Among other services, APLA-funded programs provided AIDS-afflicted individuals with supplemental income, disability insurance, help in applying for public programs, and counseling. It survived by raising small amounts of money from benefits held at bars catering to gays and other gay gathering places.

"We worked like crazy people,"[9] Misenhimer said, describing workdays that routinely extended to sixteen hours or more. Within the year, Misenhimer knew that he would not return to Xerox. He accepted the position of APLA executive director. It was in this capacity that, early in 1985, he contacted Taylor's publicist, Chen Sam, seeking to recruit her boss to cochair the world's first major AIDS fund-raiser. Named "Commitment to Life," the APLA charitable event was slated for Los Angeles in September 1985.

In explaining why he had decided to ask Taylor, Misenhimer later told *Vanity Fair*, "We needed a big event to raise money. . . . There are three big draws in the world: Elizabeth II, the Pope, and Elizabeth Taylor."[10]

In agreeing to Misenhimer's request, Taylor realized the possibilities. She recognized that she had the contacts and the clout to open doors and reach people who could make a difference. It was commonplace in Hollywood for film stars to accept honorary positions in charitable organizations, but Taylor didn't feel that this would make suitable use of her considerable interpersonal talents. She decided that if she was going to participate, she would actually do the work. Given the association with homosexuality, AIDS was a tough challenge for fund-raising. For the effort to be successful, she was the one who was going to have to make the phone calls. She would personally have to twist arms.

Taylor said that many big-name stars said no, they didn't want to be associated with this cause. They wouldn't even come to the gala for fear of how their presence might affect how they were perceived. "I realized that this town, of all towns, was basically homophobic, even though, without homosexuals, there would be no Hollywood, no show business!" Taylor said.[11]

Not everyone said no. Taylor convinced a handful of close friends, marquee-name Hollywood celebrities, to help her overcome the stigma associated with AIDS. Among those who took the plunge and became engaged in planning the event were her cohost, Burt Reynolds, along with Cindy Lauper, Shirley MacLaine, Sammy Davis Jr., Carol Burnett, Joan Rivers, and Rod Stewart.[12] In going public with their support, they contributed to the success of the first APLA Commitment to Life gala.

On September 19, 1985, Elizabeth Taylor and the evening's honoree, Betty Ford, joined a throng of twenty-five hundred formally attired benefactors in an overflowing ballroom of LA's Bonaventure Hotel.[13] Those who stayed to the very end got their money's worth. The evening lasted six hours and required three stages to accommodate all of the performances. President Ronald Reagan sent a congratulatory message. The unapologetic evening of Southern California glitz raised a previously unimaginable bonanza of $1.3 million for the expansion of APLA's community service activities.

Michael and Cindy Gottlieb were among those attending the Commitment to Life gala. Since their escapade at UCLA Medical Center, Taylor had called Gottlieb on several occasions seeking his advice on AIDS advocacy. Kathy Petersilie remembered Taylor calling the lab. Either she or Gottlieb's administrative assistant, Jay Theodore, would answer the phone and share a friendly word or two with the actress before trying to locate Gottlieb. Petersilie said that the inventive Theodore was so enamored of Taylor that he drew upon his talent for mimicry to imitate her calling to speak with his boss.

Cindy Gottlieb said that Taylor also phoned Michael at home. Gottlieb remembered one of Taylor's calls in particular. One morning early in 1986, he was getting ready to go to work. He was halfway out the door and, for reasons he could not remember, in a wicked mood. The phone rang and, without thinking, he gruffly answered, "Yes." At first he heard only silence on the other end of the line. Then a woman's voice that he instantly recognized as Taylor's asked him in a teasing manner, "Could you possibly be angry with me?"

Gottlieb became an occasional visitor at the Taylor home and got to know her staff. "Everything went through her secretary Roger [Wall],"[14] he said. There also was an English girl named "Liz" who did the cooking and kept things organized. He remembered the ranch-style house—which Taylor is said to have bought on first sight[15]—as being surprisingly modest. Although the home was professionally decorated throughout by Waldo Fernandez in his signature white upholstery, Gottlieb said, "It had a homey, comfortable feel. There was a lot of original art on the walls." He remembered particularly enjoying the opportunity to study at length a pair of impressionistic Pissarro oil paintings that hung over the sofa.

Cindy Gottlieb recalled speaking with Taylor on a few occasions. One was a private memorial service for Rock Hudson held in Beverly Hills. "Elizabeth was there, and that was the first time I met her in person," Cindy said. "She was quite beautiful and very petite, and she had very violet eyes. I spoke with her, just small talk. There was something very big and shiny around her neck and on her hand. I was just kind of awestruck being in her presence. And that Christmas we received a blanket from her, from some fancy milliner in Beverly Hills. It was lavender, a throw blanket, and it had embroidered, 'To Cindy and Michael. Love, Elizabeth.'"

The striking success of the Commitment to Life gala put Elizabeth Taylor in the forefront of a small rank of noteworthy individuals willing to speak out on behalf of the stigmatized disease. The event was a public declaration of her dedication to AIDS and proof of her talents as a spokesperson and fund-raiser.

She already had determined where she would go from there. Michael Gottlieb had approached her with an opportunity that arose during Rock Hudson's hospitalization. Hudson's money manager and accountant, Wally Sheft, had buttonholed Gottlieb in front of the medical center's tenth floor elevators and told Gottlieb that Hudson wanted to donate a quarter million dollars to fight AIDS. The money was to come from Hudson's share of future royalties he expected to earn from having collaborated on his biography with the author Sara Davidson. He wished to entrust the bequest to Gottlieb to be used in whatever AIDS-related activities Gottlieb thought best.

Thus, the gift was somewhat ambiguous. It wasn't cash in hand. Rather, it was a promise of cash to come . . . a gift but not quite a gift. Gottlieb was grateful to Sheft for his role in securing the promise of funding but admittedly had little savvy about how to manage Hudson's largess. His first thought was to direct the promised funds to UCLA. However, he felt the attitude of UCLA's leadership had been dismissive of what he'd been trying to do and obstinately slow in responding to his requests for space and personnel to expand AIDS research. He did not believe that would change anytime soon.

On further consideration, Gottlieb recognized that the Hudson gift afforded him the opportunity to do something bigger than simply handing over a check to UCLA. The bequest provided a starting point to help address the need for funding of AIDS research, the lack of which continued to plague progress in understanding and fighting the disease. Gottlieb decided to create a national AIDS research foundation. The foundation would develop an infrastructure for evaluating grant proposals proffered by AIDS researchers and fund the most meritorious ideas for advancing knowledge of disease mechanisms, improving diagnosis, and bettering the effectiveness of treatment.

Gottlieb gathered together a group of community leaders whom he knew personally and appointed them members of an ad hoc board of directors for what he imagined would become the new foundation. The group met in a suite of law offices in Century City and incorporated as the National AIDS Research Foundation (NARF). "There wasn't anything like that, and since the Rock Hudson event was such a pivotal event, we thought that it would be a good focal point to begin raising private monies for AIDS research." Gottlieb proposed to the board that they hire as NARF executive director Bill Misenhimer. Gottlieb knew Misenhimer from serving on the board of APLA and admired his commitment. He also had an intimation that Misenhimer felt "burned out" after several years of long, stressful days at APLA. The board agreed, and Misenhimer signed on as executive director.

The board's next consideration was how to successfully raise additional funds. The Hudson largess would take NARF only so far. The organization needed a recognizable spokesperson around whom a fund-raising effort could be developed to imprint the foundation on the public consciousness. Who better than Elizabeth Taylor?

Gottlieb sealed the deal over dinner one evening in West Los Angeles. Taylor chose the restaurant, a small, quiet bistro named St. Michel, where there were only a few tables and she knew the chef. Bill Misenhimer and Chen Sam completed the foursome in a quiet corner of the restaurant. Gottlieb explained to Taylor his belief that this was their moment. Rock's donation had afforded them a special opportunity to establish something meaningful in support of AIDS research. He didn't need to do much convincing; Taylor eagerly agreed.

Gottlieb said, "We were an unlikely group: a doctor who'd spent his life in laboratories; Bill [Misenhimer], a Xerox executive turned activist, who was openly gay; and the greatest living movie star in the world. But that night it all gelled. We were like kids, co-conspirators. We sat there saying, 'We must do something!'"[16]

In a 1992 *Vanity Fair* interview, Taylor added her thoughts concerning the evening's events: "We decided that night we were going to make a difference. Goddamn, we would."[17]

Much as had occurred with Gottlieb's 1981 NEJM publication describing AIDS, the unmistakable smell of an impending windfall lured interested parties who had not been involved in the formation of NARF to express their interest in the new foundation. Gottlieb began to feel pressure to do something on a grander scale. In particular, there were voices within his inner circle urging him to consider merging NARF with the AIDS Medical Foundation (AMF) that Dr. Mathilde Krim had established in New York City. Like NARF, AMF was intended to bolster AIDS research by awarding research grants and already had begun to make funding commitments to investigators.

Twenty-one years Gottlieb's senior, Mathilde Galland was born in 1926, in Como, Italy. She was awarded a doctorate in biology from the University of Geneva in 1953. While a student at the university, she attached herself to a small group of Palestinian Jews who were studying in Geneva at the same time. Among the group was David Danon, whom she married upon their graduation. She converted to Judaism and followed him home to Israel just five years after the tiny state had declared its independence.

The marriage produced a daughter but ultimately failed amid the harshness of life in the developing nation. Rather than return home to Switzerland, however, Mathilde stayed on in Israel, moving with her daughter to the small town of Rehovet, south of Tel Aviv, to take a position as a microbiologist at the fledgling Weitzman Institute. It was there, in 1957, that she met and in short order married a trustee of the institute, the powerful New York lawyer Arthur Krim, who at that time was head of the United Artists motion picture company and later founded Orion Pictures. She immigrated to the United States in 1958 and found work in the interferon laboratory at New York's Memorial-Sloan Kettering Cancer Center.[18]

The Krims were wealthy, socially active, and politically liberal. Their generous support of civil liberties–related causes and of the Democratic Party brought them social prominence and political clout. The Krims were occasional overnight guests in the Kennedy White House and hosted in their home the after-party of John Kennedy's forty-second birthday celebration at Madison Square Garden that famously featured Marilyn Monroe's highly personalized singing of "Happy Birthday."[19]

Gottlieb first heard about the bicoastal efforts to put him and Krim together from the prominent AIDS activist Bruce Decker.[20] Gottlieb and Decker had become friends while serving together as members of the California AIDS Advisory Committee, which was appointed by the governor and made recommendations to the California Department of Health. Decker had just returned from a trip back east and reported that Mathilde Krim wanted to meet to discuss merging their foundations.[21] This put Gottlieb on the alert, since Krim had previously made overtures to him about his coming onto the AMF board of directors. He grew suspicious that the talk of joining forces was actually an effort to preempt his forming what might become a West Coast competitor to AMF.

"We were already under way forming the National AIDS Research Foundation, and Elizabeth Taylor was committed to us. So I felt that we were coming from a position of some strength, and that we could hold out," Gottlieb said.

Even so, Decker got Gottlieb thinking. "Bruce said he thought this was a real opportunity to have a genuinely national research organization. Then Bill Misenhimer said, 'You really should do something national.'" He rolled the question over and over in his mind: Would joining with Krim lead to something that was stronger and more effective than his going it alone?

In retrospect, Gottlieb thought it was likely that Krim had been in the mix from the start, working behind the scenes to most advantageously position AMF for a merger. "Mathilde Krim made a bee-line for Los Angeles after Rock Hudson," Gottlieb said. "I think quite astutely recognizing that there was money to be raised and that Los Angeles and Hollywood was now the ticket to getting more acceptance for AIDS as a legitimate cause. And of course she was well-situated to be able to make that assessment, knowing the world of New York and Los Angeles and knowing Hollywood as a result of her husband."

The Krims soon brought to the merger discussions a number of their Los Angeles associates. Among them was Arnold Klein, a Beverly Hills dermatologist who was well-connected with the filmmaking community. According to Jonathan Canno, a member of the AMF board, Klein arranged a meeting at his house to discuss how they could get past some of the issues standing in the way of the two foundations getting together.[22]

At Klein's house, Gottlieb became aware of yet another interested party, entertainment impresario David Geffen. Gottlieb initially was perplexed by Geffen's interest, but he later heard that Geffen was grateful to Mathilde Krim for having helped him through a false alarm related to his health.

Gottlieb remembered Geffen as being very direct in pursuing how he and Krim might explore merging their funds. "So there's a meeting with David Geffen at Klein's house," Gottlieb said, "during which Geffen said to me several times, 'Let Mathilde do it.' What I think he was pointing out to me was that, in that era, it was incongruous for a straight man to be chairing an organization that addressed a problem so closely associated with homosexuality. Women were considered more simpatico. I didn't get it at the time. I was on my guard. But now I see that Geffen actually was correct."

"I was saying, 'No, I don't want to do it. The [AMF] money is too small [to do something major with AIDS research]. I really wasn't interested.'" Likewise, Bill Misenhimer was very much on the fence concerning the financial aspects of merging the two foundations.

Despite Gottlieb's reticence, Geffen continued to militate on Krim's behalf. At the end of the evening, there was no resolution, so Geffen invited Gottlieb to meet with him a second time at his office on Sunset Boulevard. According to Gottlieb, that conversation quickly degenerated into Geffen berating him for his hesitation at proceeding with the merger. "He started screaming at me. . . . I'm told that was the style of many of the studio executives and film producers at that time," Gottlieb said. "He started screaming at me, 'How can you send this woman away? Do you know who she is?' This mogul was screaming at me. I have never had anyone raise his voice to me like that before or since."

Years later, Gottlieb revisited the influences that led him to decide to merge his NARF with Krim's AMF. "There was this tug-of-war going on between Los Angeles and New York. Los Angeles is a wonderful city, but New York calls the shots. The eastern seaboard is the power center, and the wealth is extraordinary. Ultimately, the pressure was too great," he said.

Money was not an issue in the ensuing negotiations. Gottlieb had started NARF on Wally Sheft's promise of future funding from Hudson's estate. NARF had yet to begin operations, so he had little actual cash on hand, but what he had was unencumbered. According to Gottlieb, the same could not be said for AMF, which had obligated itself to a research agenda beyond its cash reserves. "They were in the red," he said. "They had made more commitments than they had money to pay for them."

The negotiations had taken on a life of their own. A momentum had built up that would not be denied. Gottlieb said, "We took a few members of her board and a few members of my board, and we merged the two boards into one."

In the patois of inveterate gamblers, Gottlieb and Krim were "betting on the come": reading the portents and signs, they reasoned that now was the time for a national AIDS foundation if there was ever to be one:

Rock Hudson's death had aroused public sympathy for those
   afflicted with AIDS.
The success of the APLA gala had shown that fund-raising for AIDS
   was viable.
About four thousand people in the United States already had been
   diagnosed with AIDS.
The science surrounding AIDS had advanced far enough that
   it could be marketed to the public as being on the cusp of
   important discoveries that might lead to a cure.
Assuming Elizabeth Taylor would transition from NARF to the new
   foundation, they had a high-profile spokesperson available
   who was willing to put her name on the line.

As the merger negotiations grew more serious, Mathilde Krim flew out
to Los Angeles to interview Bill Misenhimer. With Krim's assent, Misenhimer became the first executive director of what would become amfAR.

Misenhimer recalled his impressions following that initial meeting,
"She [Krim] was very charming, but genuinely so. . . . Her motivation came
from her heart as much as her brain." At the same time, he noted that she
immediately came across as a very powerful woman. "I guess she was used
to having things go the way she wanted. . . . You don't fight her because
she always wins, and AIDS is her life."

That left one important personnel action still to be addressed. Gottlieb
and Krim recognized the importance of securing the allegiance and active
involvement of Elizabeth Taylor. The problem was that Gottlieb had not
kept Taylor abreast of the state of the merger. The momentum of the
negotiations, he said, had been tremendous. Things were happening so
rapidly, there just wasn't the time to keep Taylor informed. Moreover, he
felt that Taylor was a true believer in their mission. She would go along
with whatever emerged, whether it was NARF or amfAR. "My one regret is
that I carried out the merger without telling Elizabeth until it was a done
deal," said Gottlieb, still feeling guilty after thirty years. "She wanted to
be involved in a national AIDS foundation. She never said 'Why didn't you
tell me?' She was a team player. I've always felt badly."

Gottlieb's concerns aside, Taylor was not totally ignorant of the conversations concerning a merger. She had voiced her reservations. But she trusted Gottlieb and had been committed to NARF since the dinner at St. Michel. What brought her around to transferring her allegiance to amfAR was getting a sense of Mathilde Krim. Krim flew back to California with AMF's lawyer, Joyce Swerdlin, and board member Jonathan Canno to discuss with Taylor what role she might play in the new foundation. In her 1992 *Vanity Fair* interview, Taylor said that what had convinced her to align with the new organization was her realization of what Krim brought to the table: a personal history, dedication, and power that could be placed in the service of HIV/AIDS.[23]

On September 26, 1985, Elizabeth Taylor stood at a podium in Los Angeles, readying herself to inaugurate the next phase of her career, one that she believed would be more important and more fulfilling than what she had experienced as one of the world's best known actresses. Flanking her were Drs. Michael Gottlieb and Mathilde Krim. Facing a room filled to overflowing with media representatives, Taylor announced the birth of amfAR. She outlined the goals of this new national initiative to raise private money to support investigations into the diagnosis and treatment of AIDS. "We plan to muster the talent and energy of America's brightest scientific and medical researchers to solve the mysteries of AIDS," Taylor asserted. "This new foundation will emerge as the national organization to support research, with the staying power to attract adequate financing and resources from the private sector, and to work with the government to turn around the AIDS crisis."[24]

Taylor went on to say that Gottlieb and Krim would jointly chair the amfAR board of directors. She would be a member of the board and serve as amfAR's national spokesperson. Hers was not to be an honorary position. She intended to fully involve herself in the foundation's work. Years later, reflecting on why she was so adamant about having hands-on responsibilities, Taylor said of her persuasiveness as a fund-raiser, "I have to show up. I can't send somebody in as my stand-in. . . . I'm a great hustler, a good con artist—in fact one of the best. There are certain things only I can do."[25]

To get the ball rolling, Taylor announced that Rock Hudson—who died the week following Taylor's presentation—had made a $250,000 contribution. Another $100,000 had been received from Aileen Getty's brother, J. Paul Getty Jr. Although not announced that day, there were expectations of additional monies from the Hudson estate. As the press conference was about to end, Taylor read a brief message from Nancy Reagan, who wrote that she believed that amfAR would prove to be a very important initiative in addressing what she acknowledged was a serious medical problem.

It seemed that day as though everyone had gotten what they wanted. People who had been infected by HIV/AIDS and those who might contract AIDS in the future witnessed the founding of an organization that would prove to be enduringly successful in raising private funds to further AIDS research. Elizabeth Taylor had a new focus to her career, one that would consume her interest for the rest of her life, keep her in the spotlight, and ultimately prove very satisfying. Gottlieb and Krim came away from the day jointly chairing a new charitable entity that would become a force in the politics of American research.

Despite the appearance of bonhomie in front of the flashing cameras, Gottlieb still had qualms about merging his foundation with Krim's. His concerns were amplified when, shortly after the press conference, he received a call from a friend, David Barry, the head of virology at the Burroughs Wellcome pharmaceutical company. In time Barry, working with Gottlieb and others, would be responsible for bringing the first effective AIDS drug, AZT, to market. On this occasion, however, Barry had seen the announcement of the merger and was calling to warn Gottlieb that Krim was untrustworthy, a "loose cannon." He told Michael that he would be better off staying away from her. Barry's phone call only added to Gottlieb's angst. It came too late. By then Gottlieb had already played the groom in a shotgun wedding. "We had it all going for us," he said of NARF. "We didn't really need her [Krim]."

Gottlieb's role in establishing and leading amfAR became a significant distraction from his primary job as an academic physician at UCLA. It was yet another major stressor that eventually would take its toll. At the time amfAR was founded in late 1985, Gottlieb had been an assistant professor for more than five years. He heard the ticking of the virtual timepiece familiar to every assistant professor seeking tenure: his promotion and tenure clock. Like the infamous Cold War doomsday clock, Gottlieb's promotion and tenure clock was ticking off the days, hours, and minutes he had remaining to secure the credentials he needed to be promoted to associate professor. He had received notice from Andrew Saxon that it was time to put together his dossier to apply, then a second memo reminding him that he had not responded to the first.[26]

Michael Gottlieb was entering dangerous territory. Promotion to associate professor is the single most crucial event of an academic physician's career. The milestone is informally referred to as "up or out," since failure to be promoted and granted tenure usually results in dismissal. Universities do not take tenure considerations lightly. Proffering tenure is the university's commitment to continuously employ[27] the faculty member until he or she wishes to go elsewhere, retires, or expires. In essence, being put up for promotion and tenure is an ultimatum. That being the case, even the most accomplished assistant professor grows anxious as the time approaches for his or her promotion and tenure proceedings.

Gottlieb had cause to ponder his circumstances. In January 1984 the Council on Academic Personnel, charged with periodically reviewing the progress of untenured faculty members, expressed concerns about Gottlieb's performance in pursuing scholarly activities. In line with the recommendations of his own department's committee, the council unanimously recommended continuation of Gottlieb's appointment "with reservations." The council's particular concern was that since his arrival at UCLA four years previously, he had published only two articles of which he had been the primary author. While crediting Gottlieb for having "made a substantial contribution in the early recognition and definition of AIDS," the council noted that "he has yet to develop an investigational program of which he would appear to be the leader." The evaluation concluded, "These next two years will be critical."[28]

In concurring with the council's assessment, Associate Dean John Pierce, PhD, expressed the hope that "Dr. Gottlieb will reveal the tenacity and ability to build a research program of the kind appropriate for eventual promotion to associate professor." He asked that his concerns be conveyed to Dr. Gottlieb.[29]

By the time Gottlieb underwent his next scheduled review at the end of 1985, he had rectified at least one of the concerns addressed in his 1984 evaluation. Gottlieb now sported an impressive list of publications, for which he was listed as the lead author, in prestigious, high-quality journals. However, blighting the generally positive tone of the report was a paragraph that began, "In regards to creative scholarship, Dr. Gottlieb continues to have problems because of the tremendous diversity of activities that he [has] had to relate to in relationship to the AIDS." Given that the reviewers cited Gottlieb's active involvement in clinical trials, as well as a major improvement in publishing his research, the criticism is difficult to fathom as anything but a bias against clinical research.

Signed by Drs. Andrew Saxon and Kenneth I. Shine, the appraisal noted that Dr. Gottlieb had been apprised of these concerns. It further noted that Gottlieb had been asked to assume less of an administrative role in order to give himself the time and opportunity to pursue more creative endeavors. They concluded their report by expressing the hope that Gottlieb would be able to achieve "the kind of scholarship necessary for promotion and tenure in the future."[30]

Further complicating matters was that Gottlieb's path had been unconventional in important ways. Whereas most young faculty members preferred to draw as little attention as possible to themselves, he was an activist, frequently speaking on behalf of a community against which there was considerable bias. His junior status made him more vulnerable than would have been the case had he already been tenured. Although Gottlieb asserted that he had never allowed his ministering to Rock Hudson and his advocacy activities with Elizabeth Taylor or amfAR to infringe on his responsibilities as a UCLA faculty member, at the very least they must have diverted a great deal of energy. That he had gone his own way with Rock Hudson's promissory note for $250,000 and established a foundation outside of UCLA, rather than bringing the funding to the university, had aroused the anger of several detractors and reinforced the rancor of old grudges. These men had their eyes on Gottlieb's promotion and tenure clock as much as he did. They didn't mind waiting. Revenge was a dish best served cold.[31]

TEN

The Contentious Route
to an Effective Treatment

Gottlieb handed Kathy Petersilie the tube of blood he had carried from the clinic. The tube was labeled with a single word: "special." This and the fact that Gottlieb's clinic was so busy that he could rarely afford the time away from his patients to transport specimens of patients' blood put Petersilie on alert. "I need the results on this as soon as possible," was all her boss had said before doing an about-face and heading back to the clinic.

Petersilie prepared the sample for flow cytometry and siphoned off serum for the ELISA antibody test.[1] Clutching a cup of coffee in one hand, she used the other to add the ELISA reagent to the serum and set about busying herself with the routine batches of tests that she had started "cooking" earlier in the day.

Two hours later she returned to the blood work of her boss's special patient, unhappily noting that the contents of the ELISA tube had turned a cloudy yellow. Positive. The results of the flow cytometry corroborated the diagnosis. Gottlieb's "special" patient had abnormally low levels of CD4 T-lymphocytes and a lower than normal ratio of CD4 to CD8 T-lymphocyte subtypes. Another poor soul had contracted HIV/AIDS.

Selecting a key from a ring she carried in her purse, Petersilie unlocked and opened her desk drawer and withdrew the notebook in which she stored the lab results on Dr. Gottlieb's patients. She found a clean page, noted the date as July 18, 1985, and entered the data. It was Gottlieb's job to keep straight who the special patients were so that she could later enter their identity. He usually remembered, but she had invented a system to prompt his memory, just in case.

Noticing that her boss had finished clinic and now sat hunched over his makeshift desk in the opposite corner of the lab, she slid from the stool, gathered her notes, and, as an afterthought, removed her laboratory gloves. A good thing she'd remembered. Gottlieb had warned her about wearing gloves she had used to work with patients' blood several times previously. Years later, Petersilie expressed amazement at some of the risks she'd taken but confessed that her appetite for flaunting protocol often received a boost from a bottle of vodka she and a few of the neighboring lab techs kept in a refrigerated room across the hall.

Hearing Petersilie approach, Gottlieb lifted his head.

"I'm sorry to interrupt," Petersilie said, handing him a slip of paper. "But I thought you would want to see these results on that special tube of blood you brought me a couple of hours ago." She accented the last few syllables upward, making her statement sound like a question.

Gottlieb turned back to his desk and reviewed the numbers printed on the standard form. The values were almost universally abnormal. He mulled the ratio of CD4 helper T-cells to CD8 suppressor T-cells. Hartley's ratio was well below the normal range of 0.84 to 3.05. "Was the ELISA test positive?" he asked. Petersilie confirmed that it was.

The results of Brad Hartley's blood work did not surprise Gottlieb. His administrative assistant Jay had alerted him the day before that Hartley had sounded anxious when he'd called to make an appointment. The blood tests had been merely confirmatory of what Gottlieb had seen in clinic. His patient had developed a fungal infection encircling his anus, presumptive evidence that Hartley had active AIDS.

Gottlieb took another glance at the lab results, wishing that they'd some-how magically corrected themselves to normal values, but the numbers stared back unchanged. Gottlieb had prescribed an antifungal agent and sent Hartley home. He would have to call Hartley and bring him back to the office. It was one of the tasks that he most disliked about his work. Inevitably, the patient would realize that Gottlieb's asking him to return to his office was not good news and ask the salient question. *Do I have it? Do I have AIDS?*

Dr. Gottlieb lifted the receiver from its cradle and dialed Hartley's number. The change in Hartley's tone of voice between answering the phone and when he recognized the identity of the caller clearly evidenced that he suspected what Gottlieb was going to say. Gottlieb was friendly but brief. It was important that Hartley return to the office for further consultation. That was all. He deflected further questions pending Hartley's visit, which they agreed should occur as soon as Jay could identify an open clinic slot in which to schedule an appointment.

Finding an open appointment slot for Gottlieb to see a patient in clinic was more easily said than done. In July 1986 the assistant director of Medical Ambulatory Care Services, Dr. Frank Apgar, complained to Gottlieb about "an increase in the referral of AIDS patients to the outpatient facilities." Apgar cited concerns that the Department of Medicine's postgraduate training programs were becoming adversely affected by too large a number of individuals having the same diagnosis.[2] The department instituted a policy that limited the referral of AIDS patients to UCLA's outpatient clinics. The effect of the policy was to make it more difficult for AIDS patients to be referred or walk in to Gottlieb's weekly clinics.

Gottlieb disputed the new policy in a letter to Apgar dated July 28, 1986.[3] He argued that the department's interns and residents were lacking in experience regarding caring for AIDS in outpatients, but to no avail. The new policy stood as written.

Somehow, despite the restrictions, Jay Theodore worked the system, and at three in the afternoon the next day the clinic nurse apprised Gottlieb that Hartley was waiting for him. Gottlieb walked to the examining room door with effort. This part was never easy. He knocked, opened the door, and entered, still wondering how he might best break the news. Hartley took the matter out of his hands. Before he could even express a greeting, Hartley blurted, "I've got it. Don't I, Doc? I've got AIDS. Isn't that what you're going to tell me?"

"I'm afraid so," Gottlieb said. "I'm very sorry."

Lowering himself into a chair, Hartley hunched over and bowed his head between his knees, his eyes focused downward on a crumpled tissue he held in his hand. After a long moment, Hartley asked, "Is there anything new that would give the condemned man a little hope?"

Gottlieb had waited silently for his patient to absorb the news. He waited a beat longer before he spoke, assessing whether this was the right time to approach Hartley with a proposal. Deciding in the affirmative, he said, "I want to talk with you about that. I don't have to tell you that there is still no proven therapy for AIDS. What I can offer you, however, is a chance to help others who may become infected in the future, and possibly yourself."

Hartley made a face, knowing what was coming next.

"I'm participating in a national clinical trial of a new drug that appears quite promising," said Gottlieb. "We're already well into recruiting subjects for the trial, but the people who watch over such things tell me I can bring on a few more." He picked up a particle board clipboard bearing sheets of printed paper and held it up for Hartley to see.

"I don't know, Doc. I'm not exactly cut out to be a guinea pig."

"It's the best I can do, Brad. As I said, the drug looks very promising. What you should know, though, is that even if you sign on to the trial, there's only a fifty-fifty chance you'll end up getting the real deal. Half of the subjects get randomly assigned to the drug, and half get the equivalent of sugar pills."

"That's crazy. Where do they come off with something like that?" Brad asked.

"Well, that is one way to look at it," Gottlieb said. "But if you step back for a few seconds and give it a little more thought, you'll realize that, worst case, if you end up in the control group and receive a placebo, your prognosis will be exactly the same as it is now. Best case, you get assigned to receive the new drug. . . . If the drug actually works, it improves how you feel, and keeps you going for some yet-to-be-determined amount of time."

"How's the drug doing so far, Doc?"

"That's the thing with a clinical trial. I can guess, but I don't know. The doctors are blinded so we can't fiddle with the data. That means we don't know which treatment we're giving to the patient, the drug or the placebo. There's a committee watching how it's going, and if it looks as though the treatment is either working as it's supposed to or is totally worthless, they'll call the trial. Either way, the sites immediately stop accruing subjects, the doctors can see who got what treatment, and the researchers release the data."

Hartley closed his eyes and went silent for a long moment. "Sign me up, Doc," he whispered so quietly that Gottlieb more felt the words than heard them.

"Brad, I know how badly you must feel right now, but I think you've made the right choice," Gottlieb said. "Before we go forward, I need for you to sign this form giving your consent to participate in our clinical trial. Among other things, it says that you understand that the equivalent of a coin toss will decide whether you receive a sham treatment having no effect—what we call a placebo—or a new drug called azidothymidine, AZT, for short."

Hartley accepted the clipboard and stared at it for a couple of beats before he signed the consent form, his body language a depiction of utter hopelessness. He had no faith that this clinical trial would save him. He was grasping at a straw, just as he might attach himself to any straw that held out even the faintest possibility of survival.

According to Dr. Samuel Broder, then a senior researcher at the NCI, hopelessness was the order of the day. Indeed, he said that Hartley's feelings were rampant not just among those afflicted with AIDS but their physicians as well.

The finding that AIDS was caused by a retrovirus contributed to the sense of futility. Retroviruses were poorly understood. Said Broder, "HIV-1 was still new, and the presumption was that treatment directed at this agent was destined to fail or cause harm."[4]

Broder said that researchers fell into two camps. The pessimists doubted that a successful treatment for AIDS could be developed until the basic science of the virus and its epidemiology were fully understood. The optimists felt strongly that even though their understanding of the mechanisms of the disease was incomplete, every moment spent waiting could only result in more suffering and death. Basic science and clinical trials of potential therapeutics should proceed apace.[5]

Dr. Broder and his research group were decidedly among the optimists. He noted several distinguishing qualities of his program that boded well for its chances to identify an effective treatment:

As federal employees working intramurally within the NCI, Broder's team had faster and easier access to funding than university researchers who had to compete for tightly controlled extramural grants.

They benefited from a long and dearly held NCI philosophy that laboratory and clinical research were synergistic. Geography was destiny. The closely juxtaposed clinics and research laboratories at the NIH Clinical Center allowed what investigators learned in the clinic to inform their laboratory research. Conversely, novel treatments developed in the laboratory were, in short order, tested in patient care.

His team had extensive experience investigating the relationships between immunodeficiency and cancer. They understood the intricacies of immunology but had the mindset of oncologists. Conditioned by their frustrations in trying to find a cure for cancer, they didn't really expect to find a once-and-for-all cure for AIDS. They were willing to accept treatments that could extend life or provide a clinical improvement—any relief from the sordid manifestations of AIDS.

Paraphrasing Voltaire, Broder said that his group had adopted the mantra, "The perfect is the enemy of the good." Rather than pinning all hopes on a cure that might never be discovered, they sought to make the best use of what they had.

Michael Gottlieb first met Sam Broder at the initial conference on AIDS and Kaposi's sarcoma that the NCI had hosted in 1982 and had followed Broder's work over the years. They had collaborated on a 1984 clinical trial of the drug Suramin I(c). Suramin had shown promise in laboratory testing in blocking the action of reverse transcriptase, the essential enzyme by which the HIV virus inserts its genetic code into the DNA of human T-lymphocytes. One of the drug's virtues was that it was already approved for treatment of an unrelated condition, African trypanisomiasis, better known as "sleeping sickness,"[6] and was available from the CDC.

Unfortunately, the randomized clinical trial proved Suramin both more toxic and less effective than hoped for. Nonetheless, Broder and Gottlieb had enjoyed working with each other. Broder had especially appreciated

Gottlieb's diligence and his sincere interest in helping AIDS patients, and Gottlieb found in Broder a kindred sense of optimism about finding a treatment for AIDS.

Undaunted by the Suramin failure, Broder's research group continued to work on identifying an agent that was effective against HIV. Among the drugs they were testing in their Bethesda laboratories was azidothymidine (AZT), a drug originally developed as an anticancer agent by Dr. Jerome Horwitz of Michigan's Karmanos Cancer Center. An analog of the naturally occurring amino acid thymidine, acquired by the Burroughs Wellcome pharmaceutical company for its oncology library, AZT was submitted to preliminary laboratory testing for retroviral activity when Burroughs Wellcome investigator Dr. Gertrude Elion had the idea to test all such compounds as potential HIV/AIDS treatments.

The drug came to Gottlieb's attention in the latter half of 1984, when he cochaired a scientific session of the International Conference of Anti-microbial Agents and Chemotherapy in Minneapolis. Among the scientists on the schedule that day was one of Sam Broder's NCI colleagues, Dr. Hiraoki Mitsuya, better known as Mitch. In summarizing what Mitsuya had presented, Gottlieb said: "In the test tube, AZT completely stopped HIV replication." Gottlieb later referred to his recognition of the therapeutic possibilities of AZT as a "goosebump moment," similar to the one he had experienced in Naples when he learned of the Pasteur Institute's discovery of the LAV virus. Excited by the prospect of a potentially effective new agent, Gottlieb was determined to participate in the clinical evaluation of AZT.

Fortunately for Gottlieb, he had connections. Earlier in 1984 he had presented an invited lecture at the U.S. headquarters of Burroughs Wellcome in Raleigh, North Carolina. During his visit, Gottlieb met Dr. David Barry, then the company's chief scientific officer. Barry impressed Gottlieb as a brilliant innovator and visionary. At this time Barry was almost certainly tracking the progress of AZT through laboratory studies and mulling over whether to bring the drug into clinical trials. Gottlieb turned to Barry to get him involved.

The development of AZT was at a crucial point. Based on the information he had derived from academic research collaborations like the work on cell cultures that Mitsuya had presented and work done in Burroughs Wellcome's own laboratories, Barry believed he had a promising new drug for treating HIV/AIDS. Barry knew, however, that positive preclinical results don't always translate into an effective treatment for a human condition.

As a result, the company faced an important "go/no go" decision. The preclinical research had cost Barry's company millions of dollars. However, for a truly innovative new drug like AZT, the expense of conducting preclinical research is akin to the loose change found under the cushions of a living room couch compared with what it would cost to conduct the clinical trials necessary to bring it to market. From this point onward, each step forward would be progressively more expensive than the last, so this initial decision on whether to proceed was critical. On the upside, if AZT proved effective in clinical trials and the FDA allowed the company to market it as the first FDA-approved treatment for HIV/AIDS, the burgeoning number of individuals affected by the virus around the world insured the demand for the drug would be enormous. Burroughs Wellcome would have a blockbuster. However, if the drug failed at any point in its clinical evaluation—if it proved to be a "dry hole"—Barry's decision to go forward could cost his company hundreds of millions of dollars in direct expenditures and up to ten years of wasted effort that could have been invested in more profitable pursuits.[7] In sum, a lot was riding on Barry's decision to submit an investigative new drug (IND) application to the FDA and move forward to conduct a phase I clinical trial of AZT.

Depending on the characteristics of a new drug, its novelty, and the target disease, phase I trials usually involve only a small number of either normal individuals or subjects bearing the condition of interest—as a generalization, perhaps as few as ten or as many as forty. The focus of most phase I trials is on learning about the drug's safety in humans. Specifically, researchers wish to determine the maximum dose of the drug that can safely be administered, identify adverse effects, study the drug's distribution in the body, and measure how quickly and by what organs it is excreted. For unique agents, like AZT, researchers also may include a few outcome endpoints to preliminarily assess the drug's efficacy—whether the drug has value against the disease it is intended to treat.

If the results of the phase I trial are favorable, and the company again decides in favor of going forward, the drug advances to phase II. Deciding to progress to phase II involves a major commitment of resources. Because pharmaceutical firms do not usually own patient care facilities, and subjects with the target disease are the lifeblood of clinical trials, the drug company must now outsource some of the work either directly to academic and community medical centers or to a clinical research organization (CRO). The CRO serves as an intermediary between the sponsor (the drug company) and the subject-accruing clinical sites.[8] Phase II trials typically involve tens to several hundreds of subjects. While they may continue to investigate aspects of safety, the main focus is on efficacy. Phase II trials generally require expertly written protocols and rigorous attention to the dictates of the protocol at the clinical sites in how they recruit the subjects and carry out the trial-related interventions. If it has not already done so, the company usually will begin a dialog with the FDA during phase II. The purpose is to gain insight into the agency's perspective on the most appropriate trial design and endpoints in order to maximize the likelihood that the agency will look favorably on the company's eventual application for FDA approval. However, while the FDA advises companies on the level of evidence they require to approve a drug, the agency's advice is not binding. In the end, the design and conduct of the clinical trials is the responsibility of the company.

Assuming that the early phase trials have provided strong evidence for safety and efficacy, the company now must decide whether to take the biggest financial bite of all, moving on to a phase III clinical trial. Phase III trials are sometimes referred to as "pivotal trials," because their outcome determines whether the sponsor will have data strong enough to submit their findings to the FDA and receive permission to market the drug. Phase III trials generally involve hundreds or even thousands of subjects; may take years to conclude; and when added to the earlier expenditures, may take the total cost of bringing the drug to market to more than $1 billion. These trials tend to be complex. The choices made by the pharmaceutical firm and its hired clinical researchers at the start of a phase III trial have far-reaching consequences months to years later when subject accrual closes and the researchers generate the results.

Knowing what lay ahead, Barry agreed to add Michael Gottlieb's UCLA site to the ones he had already recruited for his phase I trial and allowed that Gottlieb could recruit up to two patients.

Despite the fact that the trial required an inpatient stay at UCLA's Clinical Research Center, intravenous administration of high-dose AZT every four hours around the clock, and a significant level of risk attendant on the unknowns about the drug, Gottlieb was besieged by more potential subjects than his meager allotment could accommodate. Thirty years after the fact, he admitted that he had "bent the rules" to admit the participation of Dr. Joel Weisman's[9] longtime lover as one of his two trial subjects. The choice was serendipitous. The man had as part of his HIV syndrome a blood clotting disorder that left him with a severe deficiency of platelets and the risk of life-threatening hemorrhage. Unexpectedly, AZT administration led to a quadrupling of the subject's platelet count. "This was amazing," said Gottlieb, "a first-hand experience that AZT was the real thing, active against AIDS."

Decades later, in writing a retrospective on the path to a treatment for AIDS, Dr. Broder recalled that in this and other early phase studies of AZT, researchers were heartened by the observation of an almost immediate increase in circulating CD4 T-lymphocytes. He noted that it was the experience working with Burroughs Wellcome and the results of the early phase research that led them to commit to moving forward with advanced clinical trials of AZT and to broadening his group's collaborations with other pharmaceutical sponsors in subsequent drug development.

Broder's research team began immediately to try various substances that had shown good retroviral activity in laboratory testing—alone and in combination—on small cadres of consenting patients. "Within a short period, we saw signs that AIDS could change from an imminently fatal disease to a manageable illness."[10]

The positive results of the phase I research led to the rapid advancement of AZT into a phase II clinical trial. Gottlieb collaborated with Drs. Broder, Margaret Fischl of the University of Miami, and Paul Volberding of the University of California San Francisco, among others, to organize the investigation. "[Burroughs Wellcome's] Sandy Lehrman put things together. We all met at NIH to design a randomized controlled trial," Gottlieb said.

They emerged with the randomized trial to which Brad Hartley later subscribed. To be admitted to the trial required that the prospective participant have had episodes of illness referable to AIDS. Each subject was randomly assigned to either the "index arm"—mandating high oral doses of AZT every four hours (1,200 mg per day)—or to the "control arm." Subjects in the control arm received a placebo—a pill with no pharmacologic activity that had been manufactured to appear similar to the AZT pill and was taken with the same frequency.

Making the right choice of how to treat subjects randomized to the control arm is critical to the success of any clinical trial. The decision is influenced by what is the best current practice and must be rationalized on ethical grounds. One key requirement is that the control and the experimental treatments be in "equipoise," which is achieved when well-informed, objective individuals, after reviewing all the research results available, cannot say with confidence that either of the two treatments is superior to the other.

Giving a placebo to subjects assigned to the control arm had its critics. However, even in retrospect, it is hard to see how the trial could have been designed in any other way. Randomized controlled trials, or RCTs as they are called in the trade, represent the gold standard of clinical research. As little was known about AZT and there were no effective treatments for AIDS, assigning control subjects to receive a placebo was the only scientifically defensible choice. While researchers could have designed a "single-arm," or "observational" trial, in which everyone received AZT, such trials raise concerns about biases that can influence the results and would have been unlikely to have had the same impact in convincing the FDA to approve AZT for clinical use.[11]

Nonetheless, Gottlieb admitted that the researchers were in a difficult bind. "The doctor part of you is saying, 'I want to break the code [revealing which subjects were receiving the drug and which the placebo]. I want to know if they should approve this drug. I have two hundred more patients who could benefit from this.' And the investigator part of you is saying, 'Gotta stick to the protocol.'"

Gottlieb was delivering a lecture in Japan when he heard that the trial's

Data Safety Monitoring Board[12] had stopped the trial early because it had observed a positive result in the AZT arm. The trial had needed many fewer subjects to prove its effectiveness than had been predicted by the physicians and scientists who designed it. Subjects receiving AZT lived longer than those receiving the placebo.

"Fortune smiled," Broder exulted in a 2010 retrospective.[13] "The randomized controlled trial showed a significant survival advantage for AZT versus placebo, together with improvements in clinical, neurological, and immunological responses . . . [and] led to approval by the U.S. Food and Drug Administration and by health ministries in other countries, with unprecedented velocity. This suddenly changed everything. . . . These successful programs provided a reminder of just how wrong prophecies of doom can be. One can only speculate on the consequences had the outcomes been otherwise."[14]

Individuals infected with HIV, AIDS patients, and AIDS advocacy groups clamored for accelerated FDA approval of AZT. The outcry for access to the new drug was loud and effective. Less than a year later, on March 20, 1987, Brad Hartley watched as his television replayed Assistant Secretary for Health Robert Windom's announcement that the FDA had given its approval for Burroughs Wellcome Pharmaceuticals to market AZT in the United States. Noting that roughly thirty-two thousand Americans were affected by AIDS at that point in time, Windom said, "Most of them, particularly those who have had a serious opportunistic infection associated with AIDS, are expected to qualify for Retrovir (the drug company's proprietary name for AZT) treatment under the approved indications."

The approval of AZT came more rapidly than for any truly novel drug in memory. In all, from the date in 1985 when Broder's group published its first article describing its laboratory research on AZT until the FDA approved the drug for clinical use in early 1987, less than two years had passed. That's warp speed for a process that normally can take three or more times that long.

Gottlieb believed that the very early stopping of the trial was not solely due to what he recalled was a real but fairly small positive effect attributable to AZT. Political pressure had been intense. Patients and AIDS advocates were clamoring for an effective agent even in the face of significant side effects. Anemia severe enough to require blood transfusions, in particular, was a frequently observed adverse reaction to high-dose AZT. Subsequent trials showing that a therapeutic effect could be achieved with half the dose somewhat mollified this concern.

At first AZT was hailed as a savior. However, one of the characteristics of HIV is a very high mutation rate related to its imperfectly copying its genetic material prior to insertion into the host chromosome. The sad fact for many AIDS patients was that HIV was a master at the one quality evolutionary theory values most: adaptability. Over six to twelve months, many patients who initially improved with AZT therapy found to their horror that the drug's effectiveness began to diminish as the virus mutated to adapt to the adverse environmental challenge posed by AZT.

Still, the AZT experience proved the point: successful treatment of AIDS was not a pipe dream. More and different drugs were needed to address the virus's propensity to mutate toward immunity. It was what Gottlieb had hoped to be doing from the start: rational drug design and testing of new antiviral therapies. The lack of funding caused by the nation's culture war had delayed, not eliminated, the opportunity.

ELEVEN

Fear Itself

By the end of 1985 researchers had learned a remarkable amount about AIDS. Practitioners had the benefit of knowing the virus that was responsible for initiating the syndrome; that the virus preferentially infected and destroyed helper CD4 T-lymphocytes; how the virus infected cells and took over their metabolism; and that the virus was nearly exclusively transmitted via sexual contact, shared hypodermic needles, and blood transfusions. Although there was still some uncertainty about the possibility of contracting the virus by exchanging saliva, there was increasing confidence that kissing an infected individual was safe. Diagnostic testing kits that could be used to test donated blood and diagnose patients in office practice had achieved FDA approval for use in clinical care.[1]

The progress in AIDS research was all the more remarkable because large-scale federal research funding remained the captive of the culture wars being waged in the hallways of statehouses and in Washington. California, then as now a frequent harbinger of cultural cross-currents, came under particular scrutiny during 1986 for the appearance on the state's electoral ballot of Proposition 64.

The objective of Prop 64 was to have AIDS added to California's list of communicable diseases. If successful, Prop 64 would serve as an enabling law that would allow authorities to enforce mandatory AIDS testing of California residents, quarantine those who tested positive, and in some cases allow for their deportation. One authority estimated in advance of the election that if Prop 64 passed, roughly 300,000 Californians would be required to register with the state. Some 100,000 of these would lose their jobs. And 47,000 infected schoolchildren would be banned from receiving a public education.[2]

Proposition 64 was the brainchild of the mercurial Lyndon LaRouche.

LaRouche was concluding the third of what eventually would number eight hapless runs for the presidency.[3] Despite his national electoral failures, LaRouche's flamboyance drew attention and support for his radically conservative and isolationist political agenda.[4] In 1985, in preparation for filing Prop 64, LaRouche pulled together a consortium of conservative organizations with compatible worldviews. The action arm was called PANIC—the Prevent AIDS Now Initiative Committee—which collected the 100,000 signatures needed to put Prop 64 on the ballot.

The campaign to pass Prop 64 was predicated on amplifying latent fears about AIDS, residing just below the surface among the general populace. According to LaRouche, the scientists whom governmental authorities had dubbed "the experts" had colluded in a deliberate and cynical effort to delude the public. Based on the advice of his own scientific consultants, he maintained that the AIDS virus was transmitted not only by contact with infected blood and other bodily fluids, but by fungal spores, biting insects, and casual exposure, such as touching and inhaling aerosols from coughing or sneezing. In his view and that of his outspoken followers, AIDS was a much more serious threat to the public's health than the government's experts had let on. These were desperate times. Civil rights be damned; they called for desperate measures.

Prop 64 inevitably became a national hot button political issue. From his vantage point as a member of the California AIDS Advisory Board, Gottlieb watched with concern as statewide and even national politicians chose sides. Though President Reagan did not take a direct stand, the LaRouche movement received outside-the-usual-channels expressions of encouragement from sympathetic, high-ranking individuals in the executive branch who favored similar restrictions on the national level. The White House was watching closely. How California voted would be a bellwether of the American electorate's stomach for federal legislation.

Southern California congressman William Dannemeyer was an outspoken proponent. That was to be expected. However, when Governor George Deukmejian, the man who had appointed Gottlieb to his AIDS Advisory Board, signed on in favor of Prop 64 the day before the election, Gottlieb publicly resigned his position in protest. Disgusted with the politics surrounding AIDS and what he viewed as PANIC's deliberate spread of misconceptions and outright lies to invoke fear in the electorate, Gottlieb decided he could no longer advise the governor.[5]

The California electorate voted down Proposition 64 in a landslide, 79 percent against versus 21 percent for the proposition, and did so again in 1988 when LaRouche gave it another try. The public had seen through the LaRouche movement's smokescreen of pseudoscience and rejected the penal policies the passage of the proposition might have engendered.

In defeat, Prop 64 served a useful purpose. It put AIDS under the spotlight. The debate over Prop 64 had revealed the fear that AIDS insinuated into the public consciousness. That fear was felt in all quarters, from West Hollywood street prostitutes to the habitués of Century City boardrooms. As might be expected, there was outright panic among those at highest risk, what some wags snidely referred to as the 4H club—homosexuals, hemophiliacs, heroin users, and Haitians—among whom AIDS was endemic.[6]

Bill Misenhimer acknowledged, "Those of us who were afraid were very afraid." He laughed nervously as he recalled a visual of his roommate ruining their silverware by washing the utensils in bleach. He asserted that this was just one example of the preposterous misinformation about the disease that was rampant among gay Los Angelinos. His own anxiety was severe enough that Misenhimer chose celibacy for an extended interval rather than risk becoming infected by HIV. Even when he returned to sexual activity, he refused to participate in certain sexual acts that he realized carried the highest risk of contracting the virus.[7]

The medical community was no less fearful of AIDS than the general population. It seemed that everyone who was actively caring for patients during the 1980s had a story about how the fear of AIDS impinged on their lives.

Michael Gottlieb had experienced the intensity of that fear firsthand. More than once, and especially when he was deep in thought, he found his index finger unthinkingly probing the small, squishy mass at the angle of his jaw. The enlarged lymph node was a reminder of the prolonged period of unexplained illness—fatigue, lassitude, and fever—he and Cindy had suffered in 1982. He had imagined at that time that he had contracted AIDS. He had been so sure that he and his wife had AIDS that they'd contemplated quitting their jobs. In their fevered, nightmarish state of mind, they'd considered moving to the South Pacific to live out what he'd imagined would be a short period of good health before the hideous manifestations of AIDS overtook them. It was Tahiti or back to New Jersey to die near his mother and younger brother, Steven, now a quadriplegic who was nearing the end of his long battle with a spinal cord tumor. In the end, it had all turned out to be a false alarm . . . at least he thought so. Every so often an unexpected tenderness where the node lay reminded him that there was still much unknown about AIDS. Nothing was certain.

Andrew Saxon recounted a chilling episode from the early years of the epidemic. He had been a visiting professor at National Jewish Hospital in Denver, where as one of his presentations he had lectured on the clinical aspects of AIDS. After his lecture, several residents approached Saxon and told him that they had recently seen a patient with signs and symptoms much as he had described. "The next day he [one of the residents] comes up to me and says, 'Oh don't worry about it. It's just something gone wrong with a hemophiliac.[8] . . . So we blew it off, him and me, because it was something wrong with a hemophiliac." The problem, Saxon pointed out, was that soon after this episode in Colorado, other hemophiliacs began to present with full-blown AIDS. "It hadn't been realized that it [HIV] had gotten into the blood supply," Saxon said. "A month later everybody goes off course thinking about the blood supply."

Dr. Robert Wolf, the intern who brought the first AIDS patient to Gottlieb's attention, told the tale of being on-call one night at UCLA hospital when he was asked to come to the emergency room to see a patient being admitted for *Pneumocystis* pneumonia. In taking the patient's history, Wolf elicited a stunning piece of information: the patient was in the habit of selling his blood to make a little extra money. He had done so quite recently at a nearby hospital. By the time Wolf informed the hospital of the problem, it was too late. The individual manning the hospital's blood bank told him that his patient's blood had been transfused into several individuals. Wolf seemed doubtful about whether the hospital had made any effort to advise the recipients of the transfusions about their chances of contracting AIDS or of the risk to their sexual partners.

Ken Shine recalled an incident that he said led to his recognition of the lengths to which doctors and nurses would go to protect themselves, especially the faculty and staff who practiced medicine at the tip of the spear. "I usually came in [to work] through the emergency room, and I saw that everyone was dressed as though they were in an operating room, with masks and gowns and gloves and caps." Shine learned that the staff had followed the lead of the infectious disease fellow. The fellow's wife wanted to become pregnant, and he was afraid of taking the AIDS virus home and infecting her. "And of course, if the [infectious disease] fellow is going to do it then all kinds of other people would do it, but we couldn't have that. We wanted to take care of [AIDS] patients, but we didn't want to scare everybody else."

In the end, after consulting with the division chief for infectious diseases, Shine decided that the physicians and nurses, the lab personnel and the radiology techs, and all the others who came into close contact with AIDS patients should treat them with the same level of isolation and precautions as they employed caring for patients with another frightening and deadly virus, hepatitis.

Shine said that once he had made the decision, the institution moved on . . . all except for him. Shine had trouble getting past his own fears about the disease. What if he were wrong? "I spent the next four months waking up in the middle of the night with a cold sweat," he said, "wondering if I'd done the right thing in exposing these people to this agent, keeping in mind that we did not understand everything about its transmissibility." Shine considered for a moment what he'd said, then concluded: "That was a profound experience in terms of trying to confront the epidemic."

Ultimately, it was widespread fear that incited action. In the aftermath of Rock Hudson's death in 1985—after the beloved actor had put a face on the disease—a groundswell of support led to an outcry for accelerated research on treatment.

In his July 22, 1985, testimony before Henry Waxman's House Committee on Energy and Commerce, Gottlieb expressed a hopeful view of the future. In closing, he strongly suggested a course of action for the committee: "In my own view, it is imperative to institute research programs for directed research for screening of additional new drugs for treatment of HTLV-III [later called HIV]. The pharmaceutical companies must be encouraged to commit resources to this task. The task must be made somewhat easier by a good dialogue with the Food and Drug Administration. Furthermore, efforts should continue to develop a coordinated system to test promising drugs in research clinics located in the cities where AIDS is so widely epidemic and elsewhere as well."[9]

Gottlieb had plans to follow his own good advice. However, being successful in this endeavor would require a much greater level of funding then he had achieved to that point in his career. Besides, he faced a major distraction: a virtual explosion of AIDS cases were beating down UCLA's doors. Even more than money, he had an immediate need for additional staff and space to locate them where they could help him conduct research and provide clinical care.

Unfortunately, as at virtually every other major U.S. research university, so much faculty expansion had occurred at UCLA over the years and so many deals had been cut between researchers and administrators as part of faculty recruitment and retention efforts that space was the hardest commodity to come by. After some back and forth, the institutional administration offered temporary use of a small space in the nearby cancer center.

In a letter dated July 5, 1984, UCLA administrator Brad H. Volkmer confirmed that Gottlieb could temporarily use the space in the cancer center. He noted that "there is no furniture available, but you may provide from your own resources any that you feel necessary, and you may also install phones." Moreover, Volkmer reminded Gottlieb, "It is understood that this arrangement will be temporary in nature, and that it will last for approximately six months. . . . Although this is only temporary, it is the best that we can do. I hope it provides a little respite from the overcrowding of your laboratory."[10]

The space proved too small to proffer any real advantage. However, Dr. Lawrence Friedman, chairman of the Department of Medicine at the Wadsworth VA Hospital and a supporter of Gottlieb, came forward with an offer of a larger amount of space at the VA. UCLA agreed to allow Gottlieb to temporarily vacate his office and laboratory at the UCLA Medical Center and move his operations to the Wadsworth VA, a short distance from campus.

His plan was to use the vacated space at the Medical Center to ensconce the new staff he needed to expand UCLA's participation in clinical trials of AIDS therapies.

Unfortunately, the space at the VA had been unused for some time. It was a disaster from the start. On his initial visit, Gottlieb found shards of glass microscope slides bearing ancient specimens from liver biopsies strewn on the floor. More pathology slides overflowed from the cabinets. Rodent droppings speckled yellowed linoleum tile. The worst part, however, was that he had isolated himself from his colleagues. Although Gottlieb spent a good deal of his time at UCLA providing clinical service and directing his clinical research laboratory, not being on-site full time placed new strains on his ability to stay current with what was going on in the Department of Medicine and the CIA.

The inconveniences imposed by Gottlieb's self-exile to the VA resulted in stresses which he brought home to his marriage. Even though her husband had proposed the move, Cindy Gottlieb saw the fine hand of conspiracy in his displacement. She believed it was Andrew Saxon's and John Fahey's insecurity over Gottlieb's accomplishments that was at the root of why they were unable to find additional research space for AIDS in the Medical Center. "[They] did not want Michael eclipsing them. He was only a junior faculty member. Who did he think he was coming in and trying to make a niche of his own?" she asked rhetorically. "They farmed him out to the VA just to sweep him under the carpet. He was completely isolated there. I was pretty outraged about it. They should have put someone else over there and given Michael space at the Medical Center."[11]

Forced to manage his research and clinical activities from a distance, Gottlieb might have been able to make do, except that by this time he had spent down pretty much all of his political capital. His circumstances were emphatically brought home to him when Kenneth Shine decided in the fall of 1985 to replace Gottlieb as the administrative director of the AIDS Clinical and Research Center. Shine mentioned in passing in an unrelated memo several months later that his action was motivated by a negative review of Gottlieb's performance by the Dean's Advisory Committee on AIDS.[12]

Shine appointed Andrew Saxon administrative director and required that

the principals of the reconfigured AIDS Center notify the California university system, the AIDS Center's chief funding agency, of the organizational
change. A letter typed on UCLA AIDS Center letterhead dated October 29,
1985—signed by Drs. Michael Gottlieb, Ronald Mitsuyasu, Andrew Saxon,
and Peter Wolf—was sent to Cornelius L. Hopper, MD, the Vice President
for Health Affairs of the University of California system. The letter was
standard academic fare: vague hand-waving with language like "need for
new types of future activities . . . a major thrust will be needed to organize
the development and testing of modalities" without really explaining why
Saxon was better suited than Gottlieb to direct the center.[13] Under the new
regime, Gottlieb was to be in charge of developing all AIDS programs other
than those related to cancer. Cancer was to be Ronald Mitsuyasu's purview.

By February 21, 1986, the directorship had been transferred again, this
time to David Golde,[14] who succinctly summarized the origins of Gottlieb's
disappointment: "Mike, you are like the Edsel. You are ahead of your time."

Shine's defrocking Gottlieb of his directorship of the AIDS Center was
particularly significant given key events involving Gottlieb at about the
same time. The National Institute of Allergy and Infectious Diseases
(NIAID) had issued a request for proposals to develop an AIDS clinical
trial network of eight institutions. The network was to consist of research
centers with the resources and intellectual manpower to work together to
efficiently design and conduct clinical trials of promising new treatments
for AIDS. Ken Shine, in his last year as chairman of the Department of
Medicine before becoming dean, approved Gottlieb's request that he take
the lead in organizing and submitting a proposal from UCLA.

According to Gottlieb, Shine's approval came grudgingly. He said that
Shine predicted that even if UCLA were to be selected as one of the NIAID
contractors, the research would lead only to multiauthor publications and
do little to advance the careers of junior faculty. Nonetheless, a successful
proposal would bring both a tidy bankroll and research prestige to UCLA.
Although Dr. Shine denied having ever said anything of the sort, Gottlieb
insisted that in a private meeting to discuss the grant application, held
in Shine's office, his department chair had predicted that if Gottlieb were
successful in bringing in the NIAID grant, he would be rewarded with
promotion to associate professor and tenure.

Putting together an application to compete for a major federal program like NIAID's offering, entitled "The Establishment of AIDS Treatment Evaluation Units," required an effort on the scale of cleaning the Augean stables. As the proposed principal investigator, Gottlieb recruited faculty with complementary expertise, gave them their writing assignments, received their contributions, and knit the pieces together so that the proposal logically explained how the sum of the parts would work together to successfully execute the research program. Gottlieb edited the contributions into a compelling book-sized proposal. Finally, he developed a budget that conformed to the amount offered by NIAID.

For his first major foray into federal research funding, Gottlieb successfully solicited the participation of an impressive group of UCLA faculty, including John Fahey, Ronald Mitsuyasu, David Golde, Andrew Saxon, and pediatric infectious disease professor Yvonne Bryson. The payoff would come to each of these individuals in the form of partial support for their salaries if the UCLA proposal were selected by NIAID.

In taking on the responsibility of leading such a large project, Gottlieb realized that UCLA's selection as one of the awardees bore some risk. Should UCLA be awarded a contract to participate in the network, it would either force UCLA's hand to provide the resources he had promised in his proposal or exacerbate the institution's chronic problem of devoting too little space and personnel to AIDS research. In short, it would require the institution to make a choice rather than simply continuing its ambivalence concerning AIDS.

In early 1986 Gottlieb learned that the NIAID's review panel had scored his proposal in the fundable range. Soon thereafter, the NIAID sent UCLA a notice of award, making things official. Gottlieb learned of the award during a conference call with NIAID. He had succeeded in becoming the principal investigator of a five-year, $10.5 million contract. Sitting by himself in a conference room at UCLA, Gottlieb described what should have been a celebratory event "as a very lonely feeling."

Gottlieb believed that being awarded the NIAID contract would surely motivate the institution to provide the space and resources necessary to fulfill the research plan he had made in his proposal. He was wrong in this assessment. He had made a number of assertions in his proposal that were tenuous at best, including some involving work to be performed by the Division of Oncology, over which he had no control. On March 27, 1986, Gottlieb sent David Golde a letter notifying him of the inevitability of the award and asking for his help with some of the outstanding cancer-related issues. Of particular note was his concern that there was insufficient capacity in Ronald Mitsuyasu's lab to support some of the laboratory testing that would be required.[15]

Gottlieb's letter to Golde quickly found its way to the desk of his department chairman. On March 31, Dr. Shine wrote Gottlieb a stinging letter, in which he recalled for Gottlieb why he had removed him from his directorship of the AIDS Center and called him on the carpet for promising in his NIAID proposal resources that were not his to proffer. Shine wrote, "In view of these changes [to the administration of the AIDS Center], the proposal which you have made to the National Institutes of Health for clinical studies poses some significant questions regarding the availability of resources. It raises questions with regard to the relationship between this proposal and other AIDS activities." In yet another hurtful reminder of Gottlieb's fallen status, he continued, "I believe that you and I should discuss these issues with David Golde, Director of the AIDS Center."[16]

Gottlieb waited about a month for things to calm down before writing letters to both Golde and Brad Volkmer, the UCLA administrator who had offered the cancer center space earlier in the year. His letter to Golde was brief and directed at his returning to UCLA Medical Center: "I am writing at the suggestion of Andy Saxon to inquire about the possibility of securing access to interim space available for AIDS clinical research activity at UCLA. . . . I hope that you can help to secure space so that I can re-establish an office in [the medical center area] that space or move CIA clinical research nurses to the new office site and reoccupy my own office."[17]

He opened his memo to Volkmer with a similar plea but finished with an admission that betrayed his worst imaginings: "I am somewhat uneasy about assuming the responsibility of this contract without having office space at [the Medical Center] to ensure its proper conduct. Please let me know if some temporary arrangement can be found while other space is identified, committed, and developed."[18]

Receiving no encouragement from either Golde or Volkmer, he sent a second letter to Golde on August 5 of the same year, noting: "It is becoming increasingly difficult to effectively organize the ATEU (AIDS Treatment Evaluation Unit) working from the VA Wadsworth space. . . . I am increasingly concerned that the space limitations threaten the successful performance of this [the NIAID] contract."[19]

Finally, on October 23, 1986, Gottlieb wrote directly to the chair of the Dean's Advisory Committee on AIDS, to "respectfully request an opportunity to make a brief presentation at a meeting of the committee," which he noted was about a "very serious matter which jeopardizes performance of the AIDS Treatment Evaluation Unit project at UCLA."[20] The committee chose not to grant him time on its agenda.

Gottlieb noted, "The response to that grant, actually contract, being awarded at UCLA, it was again not a positive response." Despite his best efforts, he had no guarantees that space would be provided to house the program. There was no evidence that there would be any reconsideration even once the funding arrived. Regardless, Gottlieb went through the motions of recruiting staff and beginning to gear up as though space would materialize at the point when it was needed. That meant not only space to accommodate Gottlieb's programs but space for Gottlieb himself. Michael Gottlieb's occupation of his office at the Wadsworth VA Hospital was to have been short term. As it happened, his exile lasted much longer than he expected. Although not for lack of trying, Gottlieb never managed to reclaim his office at UCLA.

To a neutral observer, it might have appeared that Gottlieb's bosses were sending him a message: they had tired of Michael Gottlieb and what they viewed as his incessant demands. They wanted him gone.

TWELVE

The Politics
of Research Advocacy

In 1986, as amfAR began to consider how it could best increase the pace of AIDS research, Michael Gottlieb worried that his involvement in the new foundation had the potential to become more than he could reasonably manage. He recognized that amfAR might easily blossom into a second full-time job. In his capacity as an assistant professor at UCLA, his employers expected his complete attention, and his tenure clock was ticking. Having now invested more than six years of his life in academic medicine, he very badly wanted to be tenured. Gottlieb's involvement in amfAR and how his superiors viewed his amfAR-related activities would have a major impact on the eventual fate of his academic career.

Gottlieb soon came to realize that in merging NARF with Mathilde Krim's AMF, he had aligned himself with a very powerful woman, dedicated to social justice, who had a reputation for finding a way to get what she wanted. Moreover, Krim was not encumbered by the necessity to be employed. She could focus her efforts on the needs of amfAR.

His recognition of these circumstances crystallized during a conversation he had with one of his former NARF board members, a psychiatrist named David Sanders. Sanders said, "Well, Michael, you're in academic medicine, and you have a job, and you need to make a living, and here is this wealthy socialite from New York who will have nothing else to do but devote her time to this work. You'll be gone in a year or two, and she will eat you alive."[1]

Although Sanders's comment was meant to be flippant—it invariably got a laugh in subsequent retellings—it also was prescient. Gottlieb recognized too late that he and Krim were unlikely partners. They had similar visions of what amfAR could become, but there were important differences in how they wanted to balance differing paths to accomplish amfAR's primary objective of improving AIDS research. Gottlieb saw amfAR as the means of directly addressing the dearth of funding available to AIDS investigators. His orientation was scientific, focused on amfAR's supporting independent investigators who needed seed money to perform the preliminary innovative research necessary to attain definitive federal funding.

Krim's attention was focused on how amfAR might become a major player on the national advocacy scene. Although Gottlieb was aligned with this strategy—indeed, it had been Krim's potential to make amfAR competitive among health advocacy organizations that had sold him on the merger—he saw advocacy as subsidiary to advancing amfAR's research agenda. Specifically, he did not want amfAR to lose focus or reduce its support to researchers by investing in an expensive effort to pursue political advocacy.

Mathilde Krim's approach received a boost when the new foundation received an intimation of the kind of influence it might wield early in 1986, when Elizabeth Taylor was invited to testify before Congress on behalf of AIDS research. The conclusion of her presentation—replayed on the television sets of millions of Americans during the evening's newscasts—was an impassioned plea for greater funding for AIDS research that announced amfAR's arrival as a political force: "There is much to do. The decisions you make will directly affect how many people will be educated, how many more people will be infected, and how many more people will die. Your decision will affect how much longer it will take until we can overcome this terrible threat to the health of our nation."[2]

At Taylor's request, Gottlieb had helped her write her address to Congress.[3] However, at amfAR board meetings he resisted what he believed was "mission creep": a growing diffuseness of purpose first manifested in the foundation's greater involvement in the political sphere and then, at Krim's insistence, in AIDS education. He argued that AIDS education was more the responsibility of the CDC, and amfAR should focus its efforts on the mission for which it was founded.

"I wanted it to go in the direction of funding a lot of research, small investigator-initiated research," Gottlieb said. "I was the chairman of their [amfAR's] Scientific Advisory Committee, and I organized a process to review the grants [applications]." Years later, Gottlieb agreed that the success amfAR had achieved in its political advocacy efforts had been critical to promoting funding for AIDS research. If anything, he felt that amfAR had not fulfilled its potential in becoming the political powerhouse it might have been. He realized that to a great extent his concerns about how aggressively amfAR pursued the course of political advocacy at that time had probably been influenced at least in part by worries over how much effort he could devote to the young organization.

In addition to his usual clinical, teaching, and research responsibilities, during 1985–1986 Gottlieb had had to add a significant administrative load as acting division chief. With little communication between them, Andrew Saxon left for an extended visit to New Zealand, Australia, and Singapore, leaving Gottlieb in charge of the division's clinical coverage, teaching conferences, and bedside education of medical students and house staff.

Gottlieb was in a difficult bind. He recognized that there were irresolvable conflicts between his roles as a full-time faculty member at UCLA and cochairman of amfAR. His division chief had put the thought in his head that Anthony Fauci, the director of NIAID, might not like having a foundation looking over his shoulder and that Gottlieb's participation might have an untoward effect on his contract proposal. His department chair had made it clear that he viewed amfAR as a potential competitor to UCLA fund-raising. Gottlieb concluded quite rightly that his superiors were doing whatever they could to discourage his activism in amfAR.

Given that Gottlieb had struck out on his own, it is not surprising that the university administration grew more hostile to what he was trying to achieve in the institution. Amplifying Gottlieb's offense was that amfAR had involved in its organizational structure a number of movie industry celebrities and a sprinkling of the wealthy doyens of Beverly Hills, Bel Air, and other elite communities whose denizens had traditionally been major financial contributors to UCLA's scholarly programs.

Ken Shine acknowledged that Gottlieb had reason to be concerned. He told how one day in 1986, an "extremely wealthy man" came to his office and said to him, "Why don't you want to take money for AIDS research?" Shine said that this puzzled him greatly. "So I said to him 'What do you mean? We are actively accepting gifts.' The man replied, 'Well, I asked Dr. Gottlieb about giving money for research and he said to me, 'Give the money to amfAR.'

"That was the first I had heard of his relationship to amfAR, and you're well aware that this is the organization that was put together by Mathilde Krim and Elizabeth Taylor.[4] And I found later on, whether directly or indirectly, that Michael had become the medical director for amfAR.[5] And this individual and a couple of other individuals told me that Michael had said that if they were going to make gifts, they should make gifts to amfAR, which was very disturbing. I did discuss this with Michael. I said that if they [potential donors] wanted to give money to amfAR that's okay, but if they come to UCLA, they are not to be discouraged."[6]

Gottlieb recalled the conversation and felt that Shine had unfairly characterized him as a medical director, when no such position existed in the organization. He simply had agreed to serve on a not-for-profit board, a common activity among the UCLA faculty. He said that Shine's parting shot had been to inform him that UCLA raised more private money than any other entity in the LA area. He interpreted the warning to mean that amfAR would face tough sledding in competition for local philanthropy.

The university's vice-provost also wanted to speak with Gottlieb. He called and requested that the young faculty member come to his office on the main campus. He wanted to know why Gottlieb's new organization was a "foundation," requiring separate incorporation rather than a "society" or an "association," which might better fit under UCLA's aegis. Gottlieb had never even met the vice-provost, and the question, on first reflection, seemed to come from left field. On further consideration, however, Gottlieb saw it as an omen: "That was a sign that UCLA might have been warming up to the idea of private money. They were taken aback when a supposedly loyal faculty member decided to form a legal entity rather than bring it to UCLA."

Learning that a member of the faculty was diverting philanthropic funds away from his institution would arouse the ire of any administrative leader of a research university. After all, philanthropy is a major source of oper-

ational revenue for public institutions. It is one of the things that sepa-
rates public institutions from for-profit private ones. University deans and
presidents are often selected for their aptitude as fund-raisers. Gottlieb's
directing valued donors away from UCLA was bound to further alienate his
soon-to-be dean department chair, with whom he'd already had a number of negative interactions. However, it seems that Gottlieb had decided
that the money donated by Rock Hudson was where he would draw his
line in the sand. It was a matter of principle, worth risking his superiors'
inevitable ire.

Although he admitted that setting up a foundation was "an act of trea-
son," Gottlieb argued that it was a response to UCLA's being unappreciative
of his worth, of failing to step up and take advantage of the leadership opportunity his discovery had afforded the institution. He felt that he'd been
placed in a bind. "At UCLA, they didn't want to deal with the patients and
the politics of AIDS," he said. "But they wanted the money associated with
AIDS, and so founding an organization that was going to be giving funds to
the most worthy applicants was not something that they were interested
in. They would have liked to have used AIDS as a vehicle to raise monies
for UCLA-based research."

Gottlieb wondered aloud whether much of anything would have been
done had he brought the Hudson bequest to UCLA. He decided that no
UCLA decision maker had shown genuine support for advancing the cause
of AIDS in the institution. In the absence of UCLA establishing an AIDS
institute or some other formal home for AIDS clinical care and research, as
others had done,[7] he believed the money would have gone to uses unrelated
to the purposes that Rock Hudson had intended.

The early successes of amfAR in achieving congressional recognition,
bringing credible people to its cause, and receiving a robust response to
its initial requests for research proposals helped convince Gottlieb that in
bypassing UCLA and establishing a national foundation, he had chosen
the right path, and it enhanced his faith in amfAR's future. He put aside
his doubts about the merger and ignored his premonitions about how
amfAR might impact his own career. He lined up behind the objectives of
the new foundation.

The leadership of amfAR had been successful in wooing Hollywood's moneyed and powerful to lend their support to the venture. The names of an impressive array of Hollywood royalty graced amfAR's letterhead. In addition to Elizabeth Taylor, the board of directors boasted songwriter Burt Bacharach; actors Warren Beatty, George Hamilton, and Barbra Streisand; and entertainment power broker David Geffen. Another board member, Abigail Van Buren, adopted Gottlieb as her scientific adviser and devoted several of her "Dear Abby" columns to the subject of AIDS. Among others, amfAR's National Council included Woody Allen, Leonard Bernstein, Rosalynn Carter, Lady Bird Johnson, and Jonas Salk.

Cindy Gottlieb remembered the early years of amfAR as being very glamorous. "Not so much the meetings themselves, but there would be social events," she explained. "It seemed to me that there were a lot of celebrities. There would be entertainment, stage shows. People would get up and give talks at some of those big hotels in Beverly Hills. I remember discussing movies with Arthur Krim. He was head of Orion Pictures. That was amusing because we were both part of it [amfAR] because of our spouses." On one occasion Cindy recalled Krim taking pains to explain to her why Woody Allen's movies didn't do well in the Midwest: "We were in the Krim's brownstone in New York and had been to some amfAR event at the Met [the Metropolitan Opera House] where Baryshnikov had performed."

At other times the Gottliebs attended philanthropic dinners at which one celebrity or another hosted an evening at an upscale restaurant, and the restaurant agreed to give the proceeds to fund amfAR research grants. "We attended one dinner at a small restaurant in Greenwich Village where the evening was hosted by Richard Gere. Be still my beating heart!"

Michael Gottlieb also had very positive memories of the camaraderie that attended amfAR's inner circle. He related one memory of an evening when a group of board members had been to an affair at New York's Waldorf Astoria. It was around midnight, and people were hanging out, talking in the lobby, reluctant to go to their rooms, not wanting the evening to end. Songwriters Burt Bacharach and Carol Sager, married to each other at the time, were part of the crowd. Gottlieb said, "They had written a song for amfAR called, 'That's What Friends Are For.' We were all together in the hotel lobby and the song began playing on the sound system—it might have been Dionne Warwick singing—and we all joined in."

At an early board meeting, the directorate elected as amfAR president a well-respected public health official from San Francisco, Dr. Mervyn Silverman, who joined Taylor, Gottlieb, and Mathilde Krim as the public faces of amfAR. Within months, Silverman also took over the role of executive director from Bill Misenhimer, who was in despair over the loss of his best friend to AIDS. Once again feeling burned out, Misenhimer decided to take a nine-month leave of absence. When he returned late in 1986, it was for only a short period of time, as community relations director.[8]

Initially, both Gottlieb and Krim made every effort to be cordial and welcoming to each other. Both recognized the potential for disruption that might prove catastrophic at this tenuous stage of amfAR's development. "Things were very exciting," Gottlieb said. "We saw a lot of opportunity; it was about getting the word out."

However, it soon became clear that neither Gottlieb nor Krim was comfortable with their arrangement of shared leadership. At least on some level, there was an atmosphere of mutual disrespect that became more evident as that first year progressed. Gottlieb's perspective was that, fundamentally, Krim never was comfortable sharing the leadership. He believed that she wished he would yield to her greater seniority and experience, while Gottlieb had hoped to garner from the relationship a partner who was more deeply schooled in the science of AIDS. Gottlieb also became disaffected over Krim's view of physicians. "She had little respect for physicians who were on the front lines caring for patients, ironically calling them 'nice doctors' and 'hand holders,'" he said.

Gottlieb believed that the fundamental problem went deeper than just a conflict between two strong-willed people who were used to being in charge. He and Krim came from different worlds. The Krims were people accustomed to wielding power and expecting privilege, while Gottlieb never lost the mind-set he had inherited growing up as part of a struggling family in central New Jersey.

He remembered an evening that sharply limned their differences when he and Cindy had dinner with the Krims at the Beverly Hills Hotel. Gottlieb said that by the end of the evening he felt patronized, particularly by how Arthur Krim had refused his offer to pick up the check. "In retrospect," Gottlieb wrote, "it was ludicrous for a poor professor to pay for the meal of a studio head and his wife."[9] Gottlieb concluded, "They were in a different league. It was one I had never aspired to be a part of."

Krim and Gottlieb soon clashed over control of amfAR's core research mission. Early on, Krim insisted that she cochair amfAR's Scientific Advisory Committee. This was amfAR's key committee, charged with recommending to the board of directors which grant applications should be funded.

Gottlieb had established and peopled amfAR's Scientific Advisory Committee with some of the national luminaries of AIDS research. He had developed its procedures and recruited his former administrative assistant, Jay Theodore, and a former UCLA grants administrator, Ralph Glorioso, to organize the committee's activities, manage the applications, and execute its decisions.

One member of the Scientific Advisory Committee during the early years was Dr. Frederick Siegal, a career-long AIDS specialist who retired from practice in 2012. He had seen his first patient with what later turned out to have been AIDS in 1979—a thirty-one-year-old Dominican woman who had shown the characteristic but then not understood depletion in her T-lymphocytes—and published an article describing four cases of AIDS in the same 1981 issue of the NEJM that included Gottlieb's article. Siegal noted that numerous individuals, representing a variety of expertise, comprised the amfAR committee. "It was run like an NIH study section. Each application was sent out to three reviewers. Reviewers were not supposed to discuss a proposal until they arrived at the meeting. . . . It wasn't just immunology. We had all sorts of applications on related topics, like homosexuality and the drug culture."

Gottlieb felt that scientifically speaking, Krim was ill-equipped to participate with such an elite group in grants decision making. As evidence, Gottlieb noted that a search of her publications intimated little in the way of research directly related to AIDS. Her major contributions to the AIDS literature had been in the areas of advocacy, public relations, and fund-raising. Nonetheless, Gottlieb could not find it in himself to say no to his cochair's insistent demands. Instead, he gritted his teeth as, in his view, Krim made inappropriate statements and did her best to steer funding toward her favorite New York City–based investigators. "She wanted to study off the wall drugs that patients were using based on flimsy evidence that in the end fell by the wayside. . . . The sense we both [Gottlieb and Krim] had was one of annoyance. She didn't have a grip on the science."

The relationship took a downward turn when Gottlieb, frustrated, began taking Krim to task over particulars of her activities. A memo Gottlieb sent to Krim, dated May 12, 1986,[10] questioned several pronouncements she had made in a draft document several weeks earlier. In his memo, Gottlieb advised that he would prefer to see the word "beneficial" in place of her choice, "life-saving," and that the word "doomed" should be replaced with "seriously ill with." Most of the remainder of Gottlieb's memo dealt with what he viewed as incorrect assumptions Krim had made about the choice of no active treatment (i.e., placebo) in the design of the phase II clinical trial of AZT in which he was participating.

"Mathilde publicly rattled the sabers," Gottlieb said. "She said it was unethical to run a placebo-controlled trial of a new drug, giving nothing to some of the subjects carrying a deadly disease. She became known as the great compassionate one." Looking back, however, Gottlieb acknowledged that Krim's outspoken criticism, in concert with the voices of other advocates pushing for approval, had played an important role in hastening the FDA's approval of AZT.

By the end of 1986 the coolness between amfAR's cochairs had progressed to outright antagonism. In December Gottlieb wrote a letter to Krim that began, "I enclose a press clipping which you probably have seen already." Tongue firmly planted in the side of his cheek, Gottlieb continued, "I assume that you were extensively misquoted. If not, I would welcome an opportunity to discuss this with you in some detail."[11]

The widely syndicated news article[12] had quoted Krim as theorizing that AIDS had begun in the United States as a result of tainted gamma globulin treatments for hepatitis, which was rampant in the gay population. Gottlieb felt that there was no evidence to support such a hypothesis and that Krim's pronouncement might have dangerous consequences: "I am particularly concerned because gamma globulin is a helpful product which is safe and does not deserve the bad reputation. In addition, the many patients who have received it might be frightened by your theory. While I do not question your freedom to voice any theory, I would be concerned if this theory were attributed to amfAR. . . . I do not think it benefits amfAR to have hypotheses without evidence attributed to the foundation. Her [amfAR's] scientific credibility is at stake."

Once again, Krim ignored Gottlieb's concerns. A pattern of mutual disrespect had been established, and the course of their relationship inexorably declined.

Their differences came to a head in 1987, when Gottlieb and Krim arrived at an impasse over the issue of whether amfAR should invest its resources in establishing a series of nationwide, community-based networks to perform clinical trials of prospective new AIDS therapies. There existed a successful precedent for such networks, although they were built with federal funds on a much larger scale. In the 1960s the NCI began to fund what it termed "clinical trials cooperative groups" to scientifically evaluate the effectiveness of new anticancer drugs.[13] The cooperative groups centrally developed protocols that were adopted by their regional and national networks of physicians, hospitals, and cancer centers. The networks, which involve both university-based and community physicians and hospitals, accrue subjects into the clinical trials and assign them to one treatment or another in a uniform manner as dictated by the protocol. The recruiting power of the network and the uniformity of their protocol-dictated procedures allow for much more rapid and more accurate determination of the effectiveness of a treatment than would be possible if each individual institution wrote its own protocol and attempted to perform its own clinical trial.

Krim strongly supported the local network strategy, while Gottlieb was opposed to it. He explained that he wasn't against the idea of community physicians participating in clinical trials. "However, I thought it [amfAR] was biting off much more than it should have in terms of utilization of research funds," he opined. Gottlieb felt that Krim didn't appreciate the magnitude of the expenditures necessary to maintain the networks in readiness whether trials were being conducted or not. He saw the concept as a bottomless pit from which amfAR would never be able to extricate itself. The program would disadvantage amfAR in being able to fund the many worthwhile research proposals that were crossing the transom.

Gottlieb said, "Well, I think the bottom line is that it was a huge program with the potential of a huge commitment that was being made, and I thought that it would short-change the basic research, serious drug related research, that amfAR [had] started to support."

Krim had proposed the plan to amfAR's board as being a commitment to short-term funding that would be necessary to prove the concept. She believed that some federal institute, perhaps the NIAID, would see the value of the networks and assume the cost. Gottlieb said, "I really don't know how much money amfAR ultimately poured down that hole. But it was Dr. Krim's personal project. It was her wish, and she imposed that wish on everyone involved. . . . I'm not certain what, if anything, in the way of new knowledge was ever generated by that program."[14]

In retrospect, Gottlieb said that it should have been obvious to him that Krim had been looking for the right situation to assume sole leadership of the organization. An opportunity presented itself in 1987, when one of Gottlieb's appointees to the amfAR board, Dr. Joel Weisman, broke with Gottlieb over the issue of community-based clinical trials. Now deceased, Weisman and his medical group had prospered following Gottlieb's including him as an author on the NEJM article. Weisman was gay, and his authorship had allowed him to build a reputation in the gay community as "the gay discoverer of AIDS."

Weisman had recently hired a young HIV/AIDS physician who had applied for amfAR support to develop a clinical trials network based out of Weisman's practice. The dispute between Weisman and Gottlieb revolved around the issue of whether the private practice of an amfAR board member should be eligible to be a recipient of amfAR funds. Gottlieb argued that the conflict of interest was too serious. It was his feeling that board membership should exclude an individual from receiving amfAR funds. In his own words, "I made a stink about it."

Gottlieb realized that the dispute had made some board members unhappy, that his making an issue of it had been viewed as disruptive. However, he understood only after the fact how vulnerable the dispute had made him. With the fuss over Weisman's proposal for funding as backdrop, amfAR planned its regularly scheduled board meeting in early 1988, at which the seemingly routine item of Michael Gottlieb's reelection to the board was on the agenda. Periodic reelection was required by the bylaws, which had been largely based on the bylaws of Krim's AMF.

"Attendance that day in Los Angeles was skewed in favor of Krim's faction—board members she had appointed like Geffen and Klein and some New York members," Gottlieb recalled. Elizabeth Taylor was absent. According to custom, Gottlieb was asked to leave the meeting room while the board members discussed his candidacy. In his absence, several former AMF board members argued against Gottlieb's reelection, citing rumors from unspecified sources that Gottlieb's speaking and media activities had caused him to sometimes neglect the needs of his patients. They also bruited that Gottlieb had been involved in over-prescribing prescription pain relievers for Taylor, who chronically suffered from back and neck pain. If that became public knowledge, Gottlieb's continuation as a board member could involve them all in a publicity nightmare.

As he paced nervously in the hallway outside the meeting room at LA's Four Seasons Hotel, Gottlieb remembered feeling as though the conversation was taking a very long time. "When I was finally invited back in, one of the members told me that I hadn't received enough votes to retain my seat on the board," Gottlieb said. Angered—"appropriately so," said one board member—he immediately left the meeting room.

"Mathilde Krim orchestrated my exit from the board of directors," Gottlieb said. "It was in the style of a high-powered, organized board takeover. It was very New York, very much couched in procedure and legal terms and lengths of board service. And of course the attorneys for amfAR were [from] her husband's firm."

One board member (who did not want to be identified) said that Gottlieb's failure to be reelected was the predictable outcome of amfAR's experiment with cochairs. He speculated that such an arrangement might have proved untenable for almost any organization, and amfAR was no exception. That one chair should eventually assume control was inevitable.

That being the case, was Gottlieb's failure to be reelected the outcome of a conspiracy or simply a matter of Krim's taking advantage of the circumstances to rid herself of her contrarian cochair? The same board member believed there probably was a little of both. Although several board members denied being involved in discussions concerning Gottlieb's future as a board member prior to the meeting, they acknowledged that Dr. Krim was a politically savvy individual who would have assured herself that she had sufficient support among key board members before attempting Gottlieb's ouster. In other words, Krim saw an opportunity to do away with a recurring irritant and improvised to manufacture Gottlieb's dismissal.

Gottlieb's defeat not only ended his influence on what directions amfAR would take in the future, it also led to amfAR redacting his name and contributions from amfAR's history. For nearly thirty years, amfAR's public face has admitted only Mathilde Krim and Elizabeth Taylor as cofounders. Indeed, it has been hard to find any trace of Michael Gottlieb's relationship to amfAR. Krim's biography in Wikipedia states that "with Elizabeth Taylor, . . . [Krim] founded the American Foundation for AIDS Research."[15] Neither has there been any mention of Dr. Michael Gottlieb in amfAR's Wikipedia entry or on its Web page. With regard to amfAR, Gottlieb has been a nonperson.

Recently, however, amfAR's organizational neglect of Gottlieb has begun to change. In preparing to celebrate amfAR's thirtieth anniversary, the organization's executive director, Kevin Robert Frost, has made a start in restoring Michael Gottlieb to his rightful recognition as a cofounder with Elizabeth Taylor and Mathilde Krim.

THIRTEEN

The Making of a Radical

The nurse tapped Gottlieb on the shoulder and gestured with her thumb toward the examining rooms. It was a recurring mime. Gottlieb's next patient, Brad Hartley, was waiting for him. Gottlieb selected Hartley's most recent medical record from the precariously stacked pile of charts on the adjacent counter and hefted the thick folio with the appreciation of long experience. Opening the cover, he read quickly, skimming page after page, slowing occasionally to more carefully consider a clinical note or study a laboratory result.

Hartley had been among the lucky ones. He had been randomized to AZT during the pivotal trial that led to the FDA approving the drug for use in clinical practice. Between being on the trial and receiving it clinically, by 1987 Hartley had nearly a year's experience taking AZT.

So far, so good, thought Gottlieb. His patient was tolerating the drug well, and the benefits were undeniable. After so many years of having nothing to offer, Gottlieb was truly amazed at the difference AZT made to his patient's well-being. *A year*, he thought. *It doesn't seem like much unless you consider that without AZT, Hartley and many other of my patients might well be dead.*

Gottlieb knocked twice, then waited until he heard Hartley bellow, "Come in."

It was a pleasure to hear the vigor in Hartley's voice, which before he began treatment had dwindled to a scratchy, uncertain monotone. Although Hartley now bore little resemblance to the exuberant, athletic looking man Gottlieb remembered from their first meeting in 1982, he had put on weight and exuded at least a ghost of his previous heartiness.

"Brad! Very good to see you. How are you doing?" asked Gottlieb.

Hartley pushed on the handle of a wooden cane to hoist himself upright from his chair and straightened with a brief grimace. "Better than I deserve," he chuckled. "The miracle continues. I really do feel risen from the dead. Many thanks to you for badgering me into taking my chances and signing onto the AZT trial."

"Wonderful! Any problems?" Gottlieb asked as he shook Hartley's hand and grasped his elbow to guide him to an examining table. "Here, as long as you're standing, let me help you hop up on this bench so I can take a look at you."

"Everything is great, Doc. I really do feel blessed," said Hartley, shuffling slowly alongside Gottlieb.

Gottlieb assisted his patient onto the wax-paper-covered table, pivoted his legs over the side, and lowered him down on his back. He checked Hartley's mouth for any signs of a yeast infection and his skin surface for early development of Kaposi's sarcoma tumors. He paid particular attention to Hartley's mouth, ears, and anus for any reddened areas that might suggest early infection. Pulling a stethoscope from his pocket, he listened intently for rapid respiration and any muffling of the breathing sounds that might signal the presence of pneumonia. Finding nothing of concern, Gottlieb helped Hartley to sit upright and made sure he was stable before letting go of his shoulders. Hartley seemed frail. Still, he was free of infection and his vital organs were chugging along. Hartley was as fit as could be expected for a man whose once impending death had miraculously been put on hold.

Amazing what was wagered on a virtual coin toss, Gottlieb thought. *Things likely would have gone quite differently had he been assigned to receive the placebo.* Gottlieb felt a fleeting sadness for those to whom chance had dictated no active treatment. Still, Hartley's actions had a lot to do with his current state of health, The AZT trial had required a lot from the subjects. Once Hartley had begun to feel better on AZT, he overcame his reluctance to participate in the trial and took to the responsibilities of being a subject with exacting precision. He'd arrived promptly for scheduled blood drawing and other mandated testing and submitted required research forms in advance of the deadlines.

For Hartley, his experience as a subject in the AZT trial had been revelatory. His return to some semblance of a livable existence led him to reimagine how he might productively use whatever remaining life he had.

Virtually addicted to sex from his teenage years onward, Hartley abstained from sexual activity. He became an advocate, a subject, and a recruiter for clinical trials of other new antiretroviral agents.

Given that Hartley's clinical-trials experience had not been totally smooth sailing, his enthusiasm for participation ran counter to what might have been expected. Although he had fought off AIDS-related death, he also had suffered complications resulting from his participation in the clinical trials of new antiviral agents. One of these complications had immobilized him and required hospitalization. One day during his recuperation, while he was lying immobile in his bed, a nurse told Hartley about a ruckus occurring in front of the hospital. [The AIDS advocacy group] ACT UP was demonstrating against what they saw as the unreasonable policies governing clinical trials, the physicians who participated, and the federal regulatory structure that slowed access to new AIDS treatments. Hartley recalled, "I turned on the TV and watched. When I realized that they were just an elevator ride away, I asked to be put on a gurney and taken down there so that I could give them a piece of my mind."

In time Hartley came to view ACT UP quite differently. "At first I despised ACT UP for all of the bull they were putting out there. But I came to realize just how necessary their role was in not letting AIDS just get brushed under the rug." Hartley believed that he owed his life to ACT UP's early provocateurs, who had influenced federal commitment to drug development and accelerated access to AZT and subsequent agents that had extended his life. Although he had not previously been prone to political outbursts, Hartley embraced ACT UP's strategy of employing controlled anger and the power of outrage to initiate change. He engaged with the gay community, participating in the June gay pride parades that commemorate the Stonewall riots and provide made-to-order occasions for ACT UP's in-your-face street theater.

The AIDS Coalition to Unleash Power, better known by its acronym, ACT UP, was the brainchild of Larry Kramer, the same Larry Kramer who had written *The Normal Heart*, the play that had so engaged Hartley in contemplating his homosexuality. The intellectually prolific playwright had earlier helped found the Gay Man's Health Crisis, but had withdrawn from its leadership in 1983, complaining that the organization had been ineffective in advancing the cause of AIDS research and treatment. In March 1987, while speaking at New York's Lesbian and Gay Community Services Center, Kramer asked the audience, "Do you want to start a new organization devoted to political action?" The audience roared its approval, and just days later about three hundred people returned to the Community Services Center to help ACT UP get off the ground.[1]

In a 2003 interview for an oral history of ACT UP, Kramer recalled his motivations. He thought that the Gay Men's Health Crisis had become so structured, so conventionally bureaucratic, that it had become ponderous. Everything had become procedurally oriented. The organization had lost its way. Citing a recent antigay march on the capital building in Albany, New York, in which thousands of Catholics had participated, he asked himself why his constituency couldn't do the same.

ACT UP would be different. It would be loosely organized, nimble, focused on correcting the deficiencies of a government that had yet to design a coordinated AIDS policy. Chief among its expressed goals was to shorten how long it took for people afflicted with AIDS to gain access to experimental therapies. All was in readiness except for one thing: ACT UP needed a strategy.

Among Kramer's inner circle was Mathilde Krim. According to Kramer, it was Krim who suggested the idea of picking a "heavy," or villain, whom they could depict as the personification of what was wrong with how the government was handling the epidemic. The group chose FDA Commissioner Frank Young to be the heavy. On March 24, 1987, Kramer published ACT UP's manifesto in the *New York Times* under the banner, "FDA's Callous Response to AIDS." That same day, 250 ACT UP demonstrators took to the intersection of Wall Street and Broadway for a coordinated action, blocking off traffic, handing out copies of Kramer's *Times* op-ed article, and shouting their demands.

Kramer recalled ACT UP's first performance of what would become a staple of the group's antiestablishment armamentarium, guerrilla theater: "I had gotten [playwright] Joe Papp to make an effigy in the shop at the Public [Theater] of Frank Young, and we hung him in effigy down there on Wall Street. Where did it come from? I think it just came from all of us talking with each other all the time. I don't know."[2]

Kramer was in his mid-sixties when he conceived ACT UP, but he successfully adapted his strategies from his experiences as a young man starting out in the movie business. He attributed the early accomplishments of ACT UP in addressing discriminatory policies against gays and people with AIDS to a two-pronged approach, in which one tine was intended to menacingly frighten and the other to politely negotiate.

> The bad cops were all the kids on the floor, and the good cops were all the people inside doing the negotiating. In the end, that's what it boiled down to. And that I learned in the movie business. That's how every successful company of any kind really works. You've got a shit executive, who fires everybody, or cuts everybody's budget. And you've got a saint executive, who keeps everybody happy. And don't think they don't talk to each other, at the end of the day, to compare notes. And that's basically what I think I was trying to steer ACT UP towards.[3]

"The kids on the floor" could be unpredictable and outrageous. ACT UP encouraged flamboyant behavior as a way of gaining attention, but not necessarily in a premeditated fashion. The group was fundamentally anarchist. It intentionally lacked an organizational matrix. In principle, committees came up with ideas that were brought to a coordinating committee, but in practice, ideas could be brought up and approved at any time and by a shifting cast of characters.

Natural targets for ACT UP's attentions were literally everywhere: the schools, the press, and naturally, the government. Given the group's early focus on New York, it was inevitable that early direct action would target the outspoken cardinal of the New York Catholic Diocese, John O'Connor.

O'Connor was hardly shy about voicing his public opposition to homosexuality, sex education in the schools, and abortion. In a 1989 speech O'Connor said, "The truth is not in condoms or clean needles. These are lies, lies perpetrated often for political reasons on the part of public officials." In promoting what he referred to as "moral positions" on sexuality,

O'Connor was aligned with the consensus of American opinion. A 1987 poll found that 78 percent of Americans believed that homosexuality was "always wrong." Overwhelmingly, the public believed that AIDS was linked to sexual immorality.[4]

ACT UP's highly publicized "Stop the Church" protest in 1989 put the fledgling organization on the map. An estimated five thousand ACT UP supporters protested O'Connor's positions in front of New York's St. Patrick's Cathedral on the eponymous Catholic holiday. In testimony to the improvisational character of ACT UP, a handful of demonstrators broke ranks and entered the church, passively lying in the aisles and disrupting the service.

Although widely condemned in the press and by leading political figures that included New York Mayor Ed Koch and Governor Mario Cuomo, Kramer considered the Stop the Church protest to have been ACT UP's most successful demonstration. "I think the most successful demonstration, in terms of what it accomplished for us, was the St. Patrick's Day thing. I remember going to the meeting after it—everybody was terrified after it, because it had been in the paper and every editorial page in town had dumped on us. People were scared, and I remember saying, 'Are you crazy? Are you crazy? They're afraid of us now!'"

The passage of time proved Kramer right. The Stop the Church demonstration achieved national notice and made the case for the loosely constituted body as a force to be reckoned with. The action was a watershed moment in bringing to public consciousness the disregard, punitive behavior, and even banishment imposed by fellow religionists upon gay men, and especially on those with AIDS. Brad Hartley's summation of how he felt organized religion had treated him could have been the anthem of any number of gay men. "There hadn't been a lot of room for me as a gay man in any of the religions," he said. "I don't believe there's a God who could make people that way [homosexual] and have them face such bigotry. It's not a choice. You're attracted to whom you're attracted."

In the process of outraging traditional society, ACT UP fulfilled many of its promises. The organization had much to do with achieving broad-based recognition of the inequities suffered by gays and mobilizing a dedicated force of people to address them. Its contribution was essential to promoting the reforms of the 1990s protecting Americans with AIDS from discrimination, establishing a federal office on AIDS policy, and greatly increasing the national investment in AIDS research.

When asked in 2003 what he thought had been the greatest contribution of ACT UP, Kramer gave a nod to Brad Hartley and all the others like him. "I have no doubt in my mind," he answered decisively. "Those fucking drugs are out there because of ACT UP. And that's our greatest, greatest achievement—totally."[5]

FOURTEEN

Le Deluge

Venice is a small, funky California village tucked between the up-scale communities of Marina del Ray and Santa Monica on the west side of LA. The town is noteworthy for its anything goes, carnival-like beach scene. The habitués of the Venice boardwalk are diverse. Ganja-smoking street youths share the surfside footpath with steroid-stoked musclemen and shapely in-line skaters waiting for their Hollywood break. Sunburned tourists jostle for the best vantage points from which to watch some of the world's most talented and outrageous street performers.

During the 1980s Robert Gruenberg was one of the Venice weirdfest's most popular impromptu entertainers. Even on slow traffic days, Gruenberg attracted an audience with his blend of in-your-face, insult humor and chainsaw executions of plastic celebrities. He continued his unfettered patter while juggling diverse, seemingly randomly chosen objects: a cantaloupe, a plum, and a throwing knife; a machete, a bowling ball, and an apple. He took a bite of the apple each time it came around. People gathered to watch Gruenberg for the same reason they attend stock car races or go to ice hockey games. During Gruenberg's hare's-whisker-from-an-amputation finale, he juggled live chainsaws. Deft as he was, the crowd still smelled the possibility of blood.

About five miles to the east, Gottlieb found himself in similar circumstances. He had a number of balls in the air, all of them vying for his attention. His mind was often with his brother Steven in New Jersey, who was dying of the indolent spinal cord tumor that over the years had painfully claimed his faculties. He was dealing with the deterioration of his relationship with Mathilde Krim, which eventually would lead to a showdown and his being voted off the amfAR board. He had spent six years treating patients with a universally mortal prognosis, all the while having to plead with a seemingly unsympathetic institution for the resources he felt necessary to improve their care. In doing so, he had alienated some powerful individuals and earned a number of detractors. Like a ship approaching along the horizon, his reckoning with the promotion and tenure process loomed larger each day. His antagonists were watching, waiting for the chainsaw to slip. Gottlieb admitted that, taken all together, it was too much for him. He was in crisis.[1]

"I was a wreck," Gottlieb said years later. "I was torn by all of this. . . . When you're dealing with AIDS, you're immersed in people falling apart and people dying, and you're immersed in dying. And they're young people. They're your age, and it changes your perspective dramatically."[2] In retrospect, Gottlieb acknowledged that this had been a very difficult period in his life and that it had stressed him beyond what he realized at the time. Overwhelmed by his personal concerns, he began to drink excessively.

Complicating Gottlieb's ability to deal with his major concerns were a number of distractions. Gottlieb said that following Andy Saxon's return from his foreign travels, their association grew progressively more combative. Gottlieb recalled one argument in particular, in which he said they had come close to exchanging blows. According to Gottlieb, Saxon had accused him of wanting to take his job as division head. Gottlieb was taken completely by surprise. That specific idea had never occurred to him, though he admitted he had toyed with a grander ambition: he'd occasionally fantasized heading up a "division of AIDS medicine" or an "AIDS institute" that would dwarf the CIA. A number of such entities had been initiated at medical centers around the country. He had never acted on the idea, because of lack of time and his uncertainty about whom he could count on for political support.

In the spring of 1986 the relationship between the two men reached its nadir. Their mutual distrust caused them to begin documenting their interactions in letters and memoranda that reflected an escalating tit-for-tat that Saxon later acknowledged could not possibly have benefited either one of them. On March 31, 1986, Gottlieb sent Saxon a letter responding to a March 7 missive he'd received from Saxon.[3] Saxon's letter had questioned why Gottlieb had canceled his regularly scheduled allergy clinic on two recent occasions and implied concerns about Gottlieb's commitment to patient care. He also chided Gottlieb about his failure to fully participate in the activities of the CIA.

In the last paragraph of his letter, Saxon asked Gottlieb to spell out the grant monies and clinical revenues that would underpin his salary for the coming year. As Gottlieb's division head, Saxon had every right to ask for the accounting. However, Gottlieb could hardly have missed the subtext. Considering the tone of Saxon's letter and the status of their relationship, he quite reasonably interpreted the query as an existential threat.

In his reply, Gottlieb questioned the validity of Saxon's concerns and pointed to his not having office space at the medical center as the source of any actual problems. The imposition of having to travel back and forth from his office at the VA hospital was the principal cause of his difficulty in keeping up with Saxon's expectations. Gottlieb wrote in his reply, "By its very nature, this factor makes it extremely difficult to interact with both faculty and fellows of the division and to actively participate in the research activity ongoing in the clinics and in my laboratory."

Gottlieb took the opportunity to remind Saxon that he had extended himself beyond usual expectations in holding together the division and fulfilling the division chief's responsibilities during Saxon's time out of the country. Receiving no reply, Gottlieb requested confirmation from Saxon in a second letter, written April 23, 1986. In that letter, he noted having followed Saxon's suggestion that he request office space in the medical center from David Golde, who had replaced him as director of the AIDS Center. The request went unacknowledged.[4]

Amid the disappointments, however, there was one very bright spot. As things were falling apart for Gottlieb in his division, he learned that his $10.3 million NIAID proposal had been funded.

The award was large enough that it rated a story in the university newspaper, the *Daily Bruin*. For a few days Gottlieb was a minor celebrity. Colleagues congratulated him on the achievement with high fives as he walked the hospital corridors. However, the award in no way alleviated the tension between Gottlieb and his division chief. By the fall of 1986, as Gottlieb planned for the funds he imagined would support a major expansion of space and personnel for AIDS research, he regretted having included Saxon in the contract proposal. Although Saxon's role was to be a minor one, Gottlieb found the prospect of dealing with Saxon in close quarters, on a regular basis, untenable.

On October 14, 1986, Gottlieb wrote his NIAID project officer, Dr. Maureen Myers, advising her that Saxon would no longer be associated with the contract. Gottlieb asserted: "This is by mutual agreement. His name should be removed from the personnel listing."[5] Gottlieb was the lone signatory. When Dr. Myers requested from Gottlieb confirmation from Dr. Saxon of his desire to remove himself as an investigator, Gottlieb wrote Saxon a letter asking that he formally resign from the contract in writing.[6] In addition, he asked that Saxon send copies of the resignation letter to his coprincipal investigators, Drs. Bryson and Mitsuyasu.[7]

Saxon wrote in his reply of October 27, 1986, that he wanted to set the record straight. He acknowledged in the letter that as principal investigator, Gottlieb had every right to ask him to resign from the project. In a manner implying that he had lost little, he said that he had no objection, but he wanted it known that it had been Gottlieb, not he, who had originally asked their project officer to remove Saxon as an investigator.[8]

As 1986 progressed, Gottlieb found himself bedeviled by a chorus of administrative disputes with members of the Department of Medicine faculty that threatened both his continuing care of AIDS patients and access to the subjects he would need to fulfill the requirements of the NIAID contract. Depressed and feeling put upon, Gottlieb reacted defensively to each fresh attack when collegial avenues of compromise might have proven more effective in building supportive relationships. Years later Gottlieb admitted that he had too often allowed his overweening sense of rectitude—what his sister-in-law referred to as his "genetic inflexibility"—to isolate him from other faculty when compromise might have served him better. He acknowledged that he had made some serious mistakes in how he dealt with various situations, which might have been more manageable if he had adopted a more collaborative approach.

Ken Shine was one who was critical of Gottlieb's manner in dealing with administrative issues, but he argued that the origins of the antagonism

Gottlieb detected among his colleagues were more complex. Shine said, "I thought he had a lot of potential and, despite the Wolf incident,[9] I thought that he could put together a program. So he began to see the patients and act as an important consultant. Then I began to get some feedback that wasn't so positive."[10]

Dr. Shine asserted that several individuals in the Department of Medicine had contacted him directly and in confidence about problems working with Gottlieb. "I was being told that he would negotiate his name on any paper that would be published as a consequence of [AIDS] research by virtue of his controlling the patients. . . . So he very quickly developed a huge bibliography. But among his peers there was a feeling that he had contributed very little to those papers. This was his pattern, at least for the complaints I received. . . . I did not take any formal action with regards to this, but I did indicate to him that I had concerns about this approach, and he argued that he was contributing to these papers, and this became an item of some uncertainty."[11]

For his part, Gottlieb denied that there had ever been a conversation between Dr. Shine and himself addressing concerns over his bibliography or his relationships with other faculty. Indeed, Gottlieb denied what he regarded as Shine's "defamatory allegation" that he had insisted on authorship, except for one instance when he had objected to being excluded. Without Gottlieb's knowledge (until he saw it in print), members of the infectious disease division of his own department had published an article detailing an autopsy series of AIDS patients, many of whom had been cared for by Dr. Gottlieb. "I simply voiced surprise that they would publish the article without even telling me they were doing it," Gottlieb said.

However, Shine's concerns went beyond the issue of whether Gottlieb deserved authorship on manuscripts written by other UCLA physicians working with AIDS patients. "It was increasingly clear that Michael was not respected by his colleagues. There were multiple issues. It was publishing all this stuff that he hadn't really done, the notion that he had divided loyalties [between amfAR and UCLA], whom he was dealing with (celebrities such as Rock Hudson and Elizabeth Taylor), and that he wasn't very effective."

"He was not a good administrator," Shine continued. "This became clear when the NIH—I can't remember the year—came out with major grants for drug testing. So this would be a number of years into the epidemic. It was very clear that the faculty did not want those projects run by Michael."[12] Feeling under attack, Gottlieb allowed his growing negativity to leak into his private life. The stresses of his workplace added further discord to a relationship with his wife that had grown tenuous. Cindy Gottlieb spoke of that period almost as though she had been an uninvolved observer, seeing a train wreck coming but unable to intervene. "They put a lot of stress on our marriage," she said, referring to Saxon and Shine. "He was unhappy with them. They weren't giving him the recognition that I thought he definitely was entitled to. Our friends from other places had such high regard for him, and why he didn't get it in his own institution. . . . The people around him were just little people. They treated him like shit the whole time. They were disrespectful. They didn't want him disrupting their little kingdoms. You know . . . academic politics."[13]

Cindy spoke fatalistically about how she assessed her marriage at that point in time: "Michael was becoming distant. He'd come home late. He'd take off his jacket and shoes and just leave them on the sofa. He wouldn't ask about my day. He'd just launch into who he'd talked to and what they'd said."

Michael and Cindy Gottlieb separated on Thanksgiving day in 1987. Their divorce became final in 1990. "I had my own circle of friends. I had seen enough. . . . I still love him. I'll always love him, but I didn't want to live with him anymore," she said.

Gottlieb was staggering under the weight of a concatenation of adverse situations affecting his professional and personal existence. However, for him, the crowning blow was the institution's repeated denial of his requests for space and other resources necessary for him to fulfill the NIAID contract. He had convinced himself that the contract would make the case with his superiors for the importance of HIV/AIDS to the institution and further their appreciation of his own worth. Although he recognized how tight space was in the medical center, to Gottlieb, it was a matter of priorities. Some programs were being relocated to new or vacated space, so why not his? Why not AIDS? The failure of the institutional administration to step up and provide the necessary space and personnel caused him to seriously consider that neither he nor AIDS was wanted at UCLA. "It was hard ball academic politics, and dealing with a young faculty member—it was really very abusive," he said. "I was bullied out."

Al Williams, a now deceased Santa Monica neighbor of Gottlieb's and a senior RAND Corporation health economist, became something of a personal adviser to Gottlieb. Williams was an Annapolis graduate who had served in Vietnam and then headed a Pew Foundation Fellowship program jointly administered by RAND and the UCLA School of Medicine. The program was specifically geared to redirect the interests of midcareer health-care providers to careers in health services research and policy.[14] One day, when Williams and Gottlieb were meeting in Williams's office to discuss Gottlieb's interest in the program, Gottlieb described the deterioration of his situation at UCLA. Recognizing that Gottlieb faced a crisis in his defiance of what Williams viewed as overwhelming authority, Williams told him, "Man, get out of the way."[15]

Gottlieb found the idea of a career shift to health policy attractive but was reluctant to give up the career he'd already built in AIDS. He began to look into other possibilities for academic employment. Correspondence dated as early as December 1984 and continuing through 1985 speaks to Gottlieb's interest at the time in a leadership position at the Brown University program in immunology. "It was interesting, it was a good job," Gottlieb recalled. "I wasn't offered the job, but I withdrew my candidacy after visiting there. It just wasn't what I wanted to do. I was very much immersed in AIDS, and Providence was a little out of the way. And Margaret Fischl, perhaps a year after I left UCLA, asked me to come down and join her as her associate chief of the AIDS division at the University of Miami, and I'll always be grateful to her for recognizing my worth and asking me to do that."[16]

While Gottlieb was sincerely interested in these and other opportunities that were afforded him by his name recognition and the relationships he'd built over the years, the piling up of adversities rendered him effectively incapable of tackling a major change like moving his career to a new venue.

He had for so long convinced himself of UCLA's potential to be a leader in the field of AIDS research that he found it difficult to imagine that he had been mistaken. Recalling how he felt in 1986, Gottlieb said, "I didn't want to start over. . . . I was wedded to LA. Cindy was wedded to LA. It was, after all, the place where AIDS was discovered, one of the major discoveries to ever come out of the place." He cited a fund-raising mailer he'd received listing the university's top fifty accomplishments. The discovery of AIDS and his name were at the top of the list.

Gottlieb did what he could to improve his state of mind. He played racquetball with a neighbor when the opportunity presented itself and picnicked at the beach with Cindy on weekends. He was soothed by long hours listening to the intricate, baroque compositions of J. S. Bach, turning up the volume to help block out negative thoughts. During one such afternoon he received a call from a psychiatrist to whom he referred some of his patients. Recognizing the music being played at a near eardrum-splitting decibel level, the psychiatrist said, "Oh, I wondered how you stayed sane."

The music helped, but more significantly, he continued the sessions of self-exploration with his therapist, Herbert Weiner, that he'd begun following the scare over his prolonged AIDS-like illness. The renowned Weiner had become the mentor and father figure Gottlieb had sought throughout his adult life. The therapy experience helped him realize that the sadness he was experiencing over his brother's illness extended to his relational difficulties at work and was referable to things that had occurred at a much earlier stage of his life. He began to understand how his childhood experiences had laid down a "fertile soil" that would nurture in adulthood thoughts, feelings, and actions that were inimical to his goals.

Gottlieb speculated that he had been wired from childhood to pursue a confrontational stance. "You go back to your early family relationships and figure out why you weren't appreciated at home. . . . It's not that you weren't appreciated but [that] your older brother [Paul] was appreciated so much more than you were. If your colleagues aren't appreciating you for what you do, no matter how hard you try, and if you're a child who was always second choice with your parents, no matter how hard you tried, the pain of what your colleagues are doing to you is so much more intense."[17]

Gottlieb felt that he had, in fact, tried very hard to gain his colleagues' and superiors' approval. In doing so, he had counted on their support to keep him going. "Perhaps they know that you're susceptible to that [need for approval]. That you're one of those people who's in it [academic medicine], in part, because you need to be appreciated. And then they withhold it."[18] Determined to get his arms around the most critical of his responsibilities and regain some sense of control, Gottlieb withdrew from the board of directors of AIDS Project Los Angeles. The organization had prospered since the success of its first Commitment to Life gala in 1985. Despite writing in his resignation letter to the board chairman, Judge Steven Lachs, that "the experience of being an APLA volunteer and board member was one of the most positive and heartening in my life,"[19] Gottlieb was nonetheless relieved to have one fewer outside responsibilities—one not related to his primary academic mission or the conflicting demands of amfAR—as he made his stretch run toward his date with promotion and tenure.

A faculty member's first step in applying for promotion to associate professor with tenure is to develop a dossier that includes his curriculum vitae and the list of his publications; the names of colleagues at UCLA and external referees from around the country from whom the institution will solicit letters of evaluation; and written statements addressing his teaching, clinical, and research philosophies.

The candidate submits the materials into what amounts to the front end of a black box, upon which the promotion and tenure process becomes wholly opaque. There follows a period of silence, usually lasting for months, during which little or no information is available to the candidate. During the silent period, the candidate's dossier is scrutinized and voted on by committees at the department, school of medicine, and university levels. Finally, the back end of the black box spews out the institutional decision as to whether the candidate stays or goes.

As his division head, Andrew Saxon was responsible for overseeing the development of Gottlieb's dossier and serving as his adviser in the promotions process. This raised obvious difficulties. For one thing, as Saxon pointed out, "I may have been Mike's boss but I never told him what to do. He was very bright and he had almost as much experience in the academic world as I did." In addition, the unpleasantness of their recent interactions cast such a pall over their relationship that neither sought the proximity of the other. The stresses grew greater when a misunderstanding between them concerning the date by which Gottlieb would have to submit his promotion materials resulted in Gottlieb having less time to get his dossier together than Saxon had originally proposed. Most significantly, Saxon openly opposed Gottlieb's nomination for promotion. The conflict of interest inherent in Saxon's being Gottlieb's promotion and tenure adviser and at the same time opposing his candidacy is hard to imagine in the current climate requiring transparency in academic procedures.

Saxon was straightforward: "Mike and I are not friends. Mike and I haven't spoken in many years. You know he didn't get tenure, right? The reason he didn't get tenure was I wasn't supportive." Asked whether Gottlieb knew of his opposition prior to submitting his dossier, Saxon said that he did not recall their directly discussing his sentiments about Gottlieb's promotion, but because the institution required it, they undoubtedly must have done so.

On August 11, 1986, Gottlieb provided Saxon with a list of the names and addresses of individuals from whom he wished the institution to solicit letters of evaluation.[20] The list was an impressive one, representing a stellar sampling of those who had established themselves in the academics of AIDS. Gottlieb asked that the institution seek letters of evaluation from such notables as Samuel Broder and Anthony Fauci of the NIH; Nobel Prize winner Luc Montagnier; and numerous deans, department heads, and professors from UCLA and around the country.

Gottlieb submitted his dossier to his departmental promotion and tenure committee, a standing committee of the Department of Medicine comprised of tenured faculty members who serve on the committee for a specified number of years. Obtaining approval by his departmental committee was the essential first hurdle Gottlieb had to clear to have a reasonable chance of achieving promotion and tenure.

The departmental committee reviewed Gottlieb's dossier sometime in late 1986 or early 1987. Citing confidentiality concerns, UCLA rebuffed efforts to access Dr. Gottlieb's promotion and tenure file. Thus the full composition of the committee and the specifics of their deliberations remain veiled. The outcome was a vote to deny Gottlieb promotion to associate professor and thereby refuse him tenure.

Several individuals were willing to speak about the committee's considerations. Andrew Saxon was a committee member: "He [Gottlieb] was very bright and he was a good guy, but he got suckered by the entertainment [industry]. You know, the Rock Hudson thing and Elizabeth Taylor stuff. He got suckered by them. The other thing was that there were a fair number of complaints to me and probably to others by people saying, 'Well, he thinks it's his disease and it's impossible collaborating with him.' You can do that with a small disease, a rare one, but it [HIV/AIDS] got very big, very quick." When asked for an example, Saxon recalled an infectious disease doctor who had phoned him to complain that despite HIV/AIDS being an infectious disease, Gottlieb insisted that to get access to the patients, the doctor would have to collaborate with him.

"It was like hawks," Saxon said, "You know how they bite their food and then cover up with their wings and say, 'It's my food.' It was just too big to hold onto, and he pissed off a lot of faculty."

What did Saxon mean by "a lot?" "There were some," Saxon replied. "I can't really tell you how many."

Could jealousy have had a role in generating antagonism toward Gottlieb? Were Saxon and the other faculty members opposed to his promotion truly concerned about the level of Gottlieb's academic accomplishments, or did envy of his renown, glamorous travel, and intimacy with celebrities negatively influence their perceptions?

Saxon said, "I didn't see any jealousy, but there might have been. In hindsight it might've been expected. You know, here's this young squirt getting all this attention."

His motivation for opposing Gottlieb's nomination was of concern to at least one member of the promotions and tenure committee. In 1986 Dr. Martin Shapiro was a newly tenured associate professor. He is still on the faculty and for many years has been the chief of UCLA's Division of General Internal Medicine. Saxon said, "I do remember being grilled, I mean grilled by the [now] head of general internal medicine [Dr. Shapiro]. Appropriately.

Whether this wasn't some kind of personal issue. I remember him saying, 'Is this something personal? Is this something between you?' You would be asked that because it's an important thing. And [I remember] my responding that it wasn't personal."

Dr. Shapiro did not specifically recall the exchange alluded to by Dr. Saxon. Rather, he remembered the deliberations surrounding Gottlieb's promotion more as a debate between two factions: those who saw Gottlieb as his own worst enemy versus those who felt he'd gotten a raw deal in a place that had not been as supportive as it should have been of a talented young faculty member. In retrospect, the distinction appears moot. A hypothetical observer familiar with the whole story might conclude that both arguments were valid and that each was directly related to the other.

Shapiro acknowledged that Gottlieb had tried the best he could to overcome imposing institutional barriers. In his view, UCLA had been less than receptive to Gottlieb's attempts to establish premier programs in HIV/AIDS and attract patients to the institution. He gave credence to Gottlieb's charge that UCLA had at best largely been exercising a holding action rather than embracing Gottlieb's efforts. "There was a lot of paranoia about the disease among the doctors,"[21] he offered in explanation.

Despite the concerns about how taken Gottlieb had been with Rock Hudson and Elizabeth Taylor, Shapiro noted that even his antagonists recognized Gottlieb was a good and caring physician. Thus, in Shapiro's mind the debate came down to whether Gottlieb had sufficient academic achievements to warrant promotion.

Shapiro paused while he brought up Michael Gottlieb's curriculum vitae, somehow saved on his computer hard drive for almost thirty years. One by one, he ticked off Gottlieb's publications during the period from his being hired in 1980 until late 1986, when the promotion and tenure proceedings began, assessing each article for Gottlieb's likely input into the publication and the value of the contribution to medical knowledge.

The exercise revealed a high level of academic productivity. Gottlieb was the author or coauthor of thirty original articles. Several more would have been in press, awaiting publication, at the time of the review. He also had contributed a surprising number of chapters to books.

Nearly all of Gottlieb's publications were in high-quality journals, including multiple articles each in such ultra-prestigious venues as NEJM, *Nature*, *The Lancet*, *Science*, and *Journal of the American Medical Association*. Remarkably for a junior faculty member, he was the primary, or first, author on twelve of his publications. First authorship is usually reserved for the individual who has carried the greatest load in generating the idea, conducting the research, and writing the manuscript. Contrary to the assertions that Gottlieb had not earned his bibliography, it is highly unlikely that he could have negotiated first authorship on any publication based simply on his controlling the patients.

Gottlieb was the last or senior author on five articles. Senior authorship is usually assigned to the researcher providing oversight or mentoring more junior individuals. For all of the other articles, he was listed somewhere among a crowd of authors. It was these articles, if any, that might reasonably have been disputed.

On the face of things, Gottlieb's bibliography reflected an extraordinary track record of accomplishment for a junior faculty member. Given that Gottlieb also had just obtained a very large contract with NIAID, he would have had little trouble in achieving promotion at virtually any major research university. At UCLA, however, whether egged on by a few antagonistic committee members or impressed by some unknowable information, the majority of committee members voted to deny Gottlieb promotion and tenure.

Without betraying how he had voted, Shapiro seemed uncertain that the committee had achieved a just decision. "Saxon was a serious scientist, and that's what he wanted in his division," Shapiro said. By way of an explanation of the outcome, he continued, "You could look at the decision and say either that Gottlieb had not sufficiently proven his academic mettle or that the committee had voted down the discoverer of the most important disease of the 20th century." The comment sounds like hyperbole, but it is not. When NEJM celebrated its 200th anniversary in 2012, it published a "Perspective" on its distinguished history.[22] From the thousands of articles the journal had published, the editors selected a handful and cited them as "Historical Journal Articles." Gottlieb's original description of AIDS in 1981 was among them.

Peter Wolfe, Gottlieb's one-time colleague in the CIA, who had been inspired to pursue a career in treating AIDS patients by a Gottlieb lecture he'd heard as an intern, went beyond Shapiro's assessment. He had left UCLA a year before Gottlieb, because being primarily a clinician had seemed to Wolfe to be a dead end in Saxon's division. Now in independent private practice, where he shares office space with Gottlieb, Wolfe spends roughly a third of his time participating in community-based clinical trials. Wolfe said, "I don't think there was anything in the way Gottlieb behaved that could explain how he was treated."[23]

Ken Shine had become dean of the School of Medicine by the time Gottlieb's case came before his departmental committee. Shine said that in his role as dean, he could have overruled the outcome of the committee's deliberations if he had wished. He refused to do so. In justifying why he chose to keep his hands off, he said, "As you know, these are blurry areas. . . . The major reason for [denying Gottlieb his promotion], I was told, was their feeling that his very large bibliography was not representative of his own personal contributions." He granted that while jealousy of Gottlieb among certain faculty almost certainly existed, it was related to resentment about the quality of Gottlieb's work and that he had accumulated his impressive bibliography only by virtue of his control of the patients.

Shine believed that the committee's decision had both confirmed the allegations that had come to his attention from some of the faculty and vindicated the actions he had taken while he was Gottlieb's chairman. Moreover, he believed Gottlieb had unfairly characterized him following the committee decision. "[Gottlieb's] media relations ascribed his failure to achieve tenure to my blocking it, which is absolutely not the case. I had absolutely nothing to do with the recommendation of the promotions committee." To which Gottlieb rejoined, denying that he had involved the press, "What media relations?"

Despite the departmental committee vote, Gottlieb was entitled to persist in pursuing promotion and tenure. He could have appealed the decision or, because he had requested that he be proposed for promotion a year earlier than the allowed maximum, he could have repeated the process during 1987–1988. Technically, UCLA did not deny him tenure. He resigned before his final opportunity for tenure deliberations occurred.

When asked whether another try a year later might have altered the outcome, Andrew Saxon was sanguine. "It would have been difficult," he decided. "It wasn't like a couple more publications [would have made a difference]. He would have had to show the faculty that he was more interested in academics. It's a balance thing. You don't say he's bad or he's good. It [the decision] wasn't universal. I wasn't supportive and when he didn't get it, he focused on me. So we did not part as friends. I don't think we ever discussed it."

Coming on the heels of his brother's death in January of that same year, Gottlieb's failure to achieve his own department's support for promotion to associate professor was the final straw. On March 16, 1987, Gottlieb submitted his written resignation from UCLA's full-time faculty, effective twenty-four days later, on April 10.[24] The one-page letter, addressed to acting chair Dr. Paul Young, listed a number of requests, among them settlement of unused vacation time he had outstanding, continued access to accounts holding present and future charitable funds donated to support his research, and admitting privileges to the UCLA Medical Center.

He was surprised at how few people took enough notice to come by and express their regrets. It wasn't for lack of knowing that Gottlieb had resigned. The April 30, 1987, edition of the *Los Angeles Times* carried a story by medical reporter Harry Nelson, "Doctor Who Reported First AIDS Victims Resigns Post."[25] The article reflected the internal strife that had characterized the relationship between Gottlieb and his department. Nelson quoted Gottlieb as saying the reason for his resigning was that he felt the institution had not been supportive of his advancement. In the end, he felt that it had not been possible to fight for the cause of AIDS within the UCLA system. To this, Paul Young responded that the real reasons for Gottlieb's leaving were that he'd had conflicts with some of his colleagues and that there had been periods of time when Gottlieb had not shown himself to be "research-wise." Despite questioning, Dr. Young declined to explain what he meant by that term.

Unnamed colleagues were as far apart in their assessments as Gottlieb and Young. One faculty member told Nelson that he couldn't imagine how an individual who had distinguished the institution as Gottlieb had could be let go. In contrast, another felt that Gottlieb had only been lucky. He had been in the right place at the right time. He had stumbled his way to success, and that success had gone to his head.

As Gottlieb prepared to exit, there was a minor matter that demanded resolution—the fate of his $10.3 million NIH contract. He inquired of the chairmen of two departments of medicine associated with UCLA—Dr. Glenn Braunstein at Cedars Sinai Medical Center and Dr. Stanley Korenman at Mount Olive Municipal Hospital—whether they would be interested in his moving the NIAID contract to either of their institutions. Gottlieb surmised that their refusals may have been caused by their wish not to alienate UCLA's new dean, Kenneth Shine.

In retrospect, it is unlikely that even if Dr. Braunstein or Dr. Korenman had shown any interest in taking over the contract, Gottlieb could have pulled off a transfer of the funds from UCLA to another institution. Although NIH grant and contract proposals are submitted by individuals, the investigators do so on behalf of their institutions. Thus monetary awards are made to institutions, not individuals. In cases like this one, where the principal investigator leaves the institution of record, NIH must make a judgment about whether the institution is still capable of conducting the research. UCLA managed to retain the funds by convincing NIAID that even without Gottlieb, the institution had the manpower and resources to fulfill the terms of the contract.

Gottlieb said, "[Ken Shine] must have been confident that the university could keep the money. He must have spoken to Tony [Fauci, the director of NIAID] and gotten assurances that if he put a responsible person—I'll put that in quotes—in charge of the contract that the university would continue to keep it." With the consent of NIAID, the directorship was transferred to David Golde.

Speaking several years later, Gottlieb tried to explain what had happened. "I saw myself as a lot of crazy people do, as somebody on a mission. . . . I decided to run with this ball and run as far as I could—that at a time when other people weren't responding in a positive way to something tragic. Horrible. I was doing what I thought was the right thing. It's a funny thing—maybe I thought there would be some deus ex machina, that ultimately the worthwhile aspects of what I was doing and had done would come to be appreciated and that ultimately something would happen."[26]

Not surprisingly, Ken Shine had a very different view. He was comfortable that UCLA had been successful in establishing a leadership role with respect to AIDS in Southern California. "I think the vast majority of people did a spectacular job," he said. "Michael, in my opinion, had a fabulous opportunity to do a great job and build a career, and I was disheartened by the fact that, you know. . . . I can only think of two appointments in my career, which I sincerely regret, and both of them were great people, but they did not maximize the opportunities to build their careers."

The tenth of April 1987 came and went without fanfare, its significance lost to all but Michael Gottlieb. Like the cacophonous glissando that precedes the abrupt end of the Beatles' "A Day in the Life," the tumult of people and events that had weighed heavily on Gottlieb's mind for nearly eight years had built to a mind-shattering crescendo. Then, with a stroke of his pen, the concerns that had so thoroughly occupied him for so long ceased to exist.

Over the last twenty-eight years, Gottlieb has occasionally taken the opportunity to order his thoughts, to make better sense of his experience as an assistant professor at UCLA. He believes the exercise has led him to a better understanding of what lay at the root of his failure to achieve academic acceptance. It was very likely, he decided, that his destiny had been determined much earlier in his career than he had imagined, perhaps as far back as the flap he had had with Dr. Shine over authorship of the NEJM article for Robert Wolf. He felt that despite what the rest of the world thought, Ken Shine had never considered him the true discoverer of AIDS. And if this is what Shine thought, it was no wonder he resented Gottlieb being sought after as the expert. He concluded, "The founding of amfAR and my notoriety around the Rock Hudson period, and my availability to the press over the first five years of the AIDS epidemic, with my name frequently appearing on the front page of the *Los Angeles Times* . . . all those things had settled it."[27]

Redeeming the Years
Lost to the Locusts

I will repay you for the years the locusts have eaten.
Joel 2:25

In 1990, three years after he left UCLA and opened a private practice treating HIV/AIDS patients, Michael Gottlieb married Wendy Gordon, a Los Angeles television news anchorwoman. Their daughter, Jillian, was born the same year.

Fatherhood was a revelation. "After Jillian was born, I dropped off the AIDS grid for several years, not attending international AIDS meetings," Gottlieb said. "Parenthood was such fun, and I was so in love with Wendy, Jill, and my new life. After much loss in my life and having witnessed so much death and destruction, having a child was a source of joy and hope. My priorities changed."

The greater flexibility of having his own practice and being his own boss gave Gottlieb the time and opportunity to participate in raising his daughter. "Sometimes parents who have hit a wall in their lives start shifting their priorities to nurturing the next generation, educating them, mentoring them, and passing along some wisdom. I was fortunate to have that happen to me," he said. Concluding that parenthood had been the best experience of his life, he wondered whether, had he remained in academic medicine, obsessed with the striving for personal achievement, he would have been able to accommodate the quieter pleasures of raising a child.

In 2012 Gottlieb attended the International AIDS Conference in Washington, D.C. It was the first worldwide AIDS meeting to be held in the United States following President Obama's lifting the entry ban on foreign citizens who tested positive for HIV. His daughter had just graduated from college.

Like her father, she had come late to the conclusion that she wished to become a physician and would spend the summer in nearby Baltimore, taking the science courses she needed to apply to medical school. Gottlieb invited Jillian to join him at the conference.

For Gottlieb, the conference was a tonic. He had been a force during the early years of the epidemic. He had maintained his currency by dint of his AIDS advocacy on behalf of the marginalized and medically underserved through his long-term relationships with the Elizabeth Taylor AIDS Foundation (ETAF), the Elizabeth Glaser Pediatric AIDS Foundation, and the Global AIDS Interfaith Alliance (GAIA), which provides AIDS education and treatment in Malawi. He continues to advise these organizations and raise funds on their behalf.

As he made his way through hallways to get to conference rooms, and between sessions, he was enthusiastically greeted by friends and colleagues, many of them dating back to the earliest years following his discovery of AIDS. Jillian was delighted to meet her father's many friends and well-wishers. Now a second-year medical student, Jillian said, "Medicine was always in our home. As a result, we had these things in common and now we could do them together."[1]

This is not to say that Gottlieb had not mourned the passing of what he had meant to be his career in academe. He did, and to some extent he still does. Nonetheless, very soon after opening his private practice, Gottlieb began to see that there were positive aspects to his new circumstances. That he no longer had to operate under UCLA's institutional strictures better fit his independent nature. He could see patients when he wanted to and, when his patients needed it, he had easier access to clinical services.

"Finally, I had a life," he said. "Starting a new life outside of academics was liberating. I had gone straight through elementary school to fellowship to [becoming] faculty without a break. School was all I knew. Advancing knowledge was my priority. It was what I was trained to do. . . .[2] In my life after UCLA, I decided to concentrate on simply being a good doctor."

Although he turned sixty-eight during 2015 and has thought about retirement, Gottlieb has had difficulty facing up to leaving medicine for good except as an abstraction. "I have a co-dependency with my patients," he said. "I've taken care of some of them for twenty or thirty years."

Among Gottlieb's long-lived patients is "Brad Hartley." Despite the worsening of chronic conditions, the AIDS-affected individuals whose experiences comprise Brad Hartley have lived long enough to see the disease that was once a certain death sentence become a condition with survival approaching a normal lifespan.

One of these individuals, who was diagnosed with AIDS in 1987 and who continues to work as a hairdresser, acknowledged that Gottlieb had made a difference: "I don't know anyone who has the passion for his patients that Dr. Gottlieb has." Recounting the many debts he felt he owed Gottlieb, he concluded that without him, "I would not still be above ground today."[3]

The man spoke defiantly of his survival, relishing the fact that he had lived with his boyfriend for twenty-eight years after he tested positive for HIV. "I've never incorporated AIDS into my life," he said. "In no way do I let it rule my life. My body decides what I do for a day. If I feel good, I go out. If I don't, I stay home. . . . There's so much shit you have to put up with. You have to laugh to get through it."

A hackneyed expression has it that laughter is the best medicine. Perhaps, but it is impossible to imagine "Brad Hartley" surviving so long without the continuous development and evaluation of new therapeutic agents. Beginning with clinical trials of the first combination drug therapies in 1992, which demonstrated a slowdown in the development of drug resistance, through the introduction of multi-drug cocktails constituting "highly active antiretroviral therapy (HAART)," the basis for modern-day treatment, HIV/AIDS patients have benefited from AIDS research.[4] An NIH Web page now lists six classes of drugs, encompassing twenty-five agents approved to treat HIV/AIDS.[5]

Gottlieb helped make possible the drug development research that has so dramatically changed patients' prognosis, both through his career-long participation in clinical trials and his cofounding of amfAR. Over the course of its history, amfAR has awarded $415 million to more than thirty-three hundred grantees and claims to have set investigators on paths that led to their development of many of the therapeutic agents now in use.[6]

There are other reasons Gottlieb is loath to stop practicing medicine. Were he to retire, he would relinquish not only caring for his patients and participation in clinical trials, but also the opportunity to help educate the next generation of AIDS physicians. A persisting irony of all the drama between Gottlieb and UCLA is that his March 16, 1987, letter of resignation from the full-time faculty asked that he be appointed to the clinical faculty, an adjunct position that would allow him to teach medical students. Year in and year out for twenty-eight years, Gottlieb has taught UCLA medical students in his office practice who are seeking to get a flavor of what the practice of AIDS medicine is all about.

Recruiting and training future physicians who want to practice AIDS medicine is a critical contribution that still faces many of the barriers Gottlieb confronted in the distant past. In 1992, eleven years after his publication announcing the existence of AIDS, the head of UCLA's division of general medicine, Dr. Martin Shapiro, and several of his colleagues investigated residents' attitudes toward caring for AIDS patients nationwide. One might think that eleven years after the syndrome's discovery, house staff would have grown used to seeing AIDS patients and their level of anxiety would have lessened. What the investigators found was surprising. Fully 23 percent of U.S. medical residents indicated that although they felt an ethical obligation to care for AIDS patients, they would prefer not to if they had a choice. This finding paralleled the results among community practitioners. When queried about the success of their efforts to refer patients to physicians in practice, 19 percent of the residents surveyed had experienced a medical specialist declining their referral, while 32 percent reported at least one refusal of a referral by a surgeon.[7]

Although no similar studies have been undertaken recently, the persistent stigma of AIDS negatively affects HIV/AIDS patients' access to specialty care. There is a dearth of qualified specialists choosing AIDS medicine as a career. Changing this state of affairs is a crucial priority. In the United States alone, nearly fifty-six thousand new cases and eighteen thousand AIDS-related deaths occur annually—this despite a 40 percent reduction in the rate of death among affected individuals. Some 53 percent of new cases are men who have sex with men, while 33 percent are primarily heterosexual. Injection drug users round out the list.[8]

Worldwide, and particularly in many developing countries, the situation is catastrophic and growing worse. Despite the initiation of a number of

multinational programs aimed at stopping the spread of AIDS and assist-
ing the afflicted, involving billions of dollars, 1.5 million people died of
AIDS-related illnesses in 2013. An estimated 35 million are HIV-infected
or manifesting frank disease. The World Health Organization projects that
roughly 0.8 percent of all the world's inhabitants aged fifteen to forty-nine
are living with HIV, 71 percent of them residing in sub-Saharan Africa,
where blood supplies remain unsafe and modern therapies are unavailable
to many citizens.[9] According to WHO, as much as 20 percent of new AIDS
cases become infected by receiving transfusions of inadequately screened
blood and blood products.[10]

Yet AIDS no longer produces headlines as it once did. In that way, it has
returned to its out-of-sight, out-of-mind past. It has been replaced in the
public consciousness by more dramatic epidemics in which the carnage
is acute and more telegenic. New epidemics, like the 2014–2015 Ebola
epidemic in West Africa, pop up periodically, most often in remote, under-
developed corners of the world. Nowadays, however, high-speed transportation connects even the most untrammeled locales, spreading the risk of
involvement to countries like the United States, whose inhabitants think
themselves protected by vaccination and access to advanced antibiotics.
What AIDS teaches us, first and foremost, is that all of us are vulnerable.

Beyond this truism, the litany of missteps in how the developed world
dealt with AIDS proffers important lessons for the future:

Ethnic, racial, religious, gender, sexual preference, and other
    prejudices should play no role in how we prepare for or react to
    the threat of future epidemics.
Modern modes of transportation and communication have made
    the world quite small. We disregard the health of the poor,
    the marginalized, and the geographically remote at our peril.
    Unaffected nations must act together, treating the rise of
    infectious disease anywhere in the world as though it were
    happening in their own lands.
Acting once an epidemic has begun is too late. Multinational
    health-care organizations must invest in the health-care

infrastructure of poorer, less developed countries, which are at highest risk for the development of infectious epidemics.

Science is powerful. Science is the ticket to gains in health. However, it requires worldwide governmental and private investment on a continuing basis, not just when crises arise.

Silence is the enemy. Public recognition, open discussion of all facets of the disease, and directed action as early as possible offer the best chances for limiting the spread of disease.

There will be more epidemics of infectious diseases. Predicting the next disease and where it will occur is impossible. Governments and international health organizations should adopt a policy of continuous surveillance and preparedness to respond rapidly and effectively. These lessons were not lost on Michael Gottlieb, whose experiences span the entire history of HIV/AIDS, from discovery to the present day. In looking back on the thirty-five years since his first publication announcing the existence of HIV/AIDS, Gottlieb was philosophical. He did not regret the involvement in AIDS research and AIDS activism that underlay his seven years of conflict at UCLA. What disappointed him was that he had not produced more new and important knowledge, that he had not fulfilled his potential in research. Nonetheless, he hoped that he would be remembered for what he referred to as his body of work—not just for the science he published, but also for his engagement with the gay community and his role in igniting public attention to the disease he discovered.

"Back when all this started," Gottlieb mused, "when AIDS had a terminal prognosis, I often said, 'My fondest wish is to grow gray with my patients.' Remarkably, that came about."

ACKNOWLEDGMENTS

A Plague on All Our Houses could not possibly have been written without the assistance of numerous individuals. At the heart of the book is the information gleaned from interviews with people who worked with AIDS and AIDS patients during the early years of the epidemic. First and foremost, my thanks go to Dr. Michael Gottlieb, who spent tens of hours of his time running down archived documents and sitting for interviews about his thoughts and actions between 1980 and 1988. Dr. Gottlieb fully cooperated with the project, knowing that I would be interviewing individuals who might contradict him and whose views would also be included in this book.

I also am grateful to a number of other individuals who afforded me their time and the opportunity to interview them. Only a handful of people who I believe may have substantive information that would have been valuable to readers' understanding of the events described in the book failed to respond positively to my invitations.

A number of physicians involved in the early years of the AIDS epidemic unstintingly shared their experiences: Dr. Samuel Broder, AIDS researcher and former director of the National Cancer Institute, now working as an adviser to a number of innovative companies; Dr. John Hanks, a medical school classmate of Dr. Gottlieb and recently retired University of Virginia surgeon; virologists Harold Burger and Barbara Weiser, married to each other, who related invaluable personal experiences concerning the discovery of the AIDS virus; Dr. Andrew Saxon, emeritus chief of UCLA's Division of Clinical Immunology and Allergy, who was Dr. Gottlieb's immediate superior; and Dr. Kenneth Shine, chair of the UCLA Department of Medicine and later dean of the School of Medicine, who was very much in the middle of the events described in this book. Other physicians whose input was invaluable to my understanding are Dr. Gottlieb's UCLA colleague Dr. Peter Wolfe; Dr. Martin Shapiro, chief of the Division of General Medicine in the Department of Medicine at UCLA; Dr. Robert Wolf, the intern who referred the first case of AIDS seen by Dr. Gottlieb, later a pharmaceutical company executive; Dr. Marc Conant, retired AIDS clinician and researcher, who provided unique insights into his patients' attitudes concerning AIDS; and Dr. Frederick Siegal, a retired specialist in HIV/AIDS medicine who served on an early grants committee of amfAR.

I am deeply indebted to several other people who are important voices in this book: Cindy (Gottlieb) Sapp, who shared her memories of the people and places associated with her former husband's work; Kathryn Petersilie, Dr. Gottlieb's assistant and laboratory technologist, who told me wonderful stories, many of which appear in these pages; and Dr. Gottlieb's daughter Jillian, who described her growing up years and her father's influence on her decision to attend medical school and help the medically underserved. Jim Chud and Peri Ribotto provided information that was invaluable to my understanding of HIV/AIDS and the period of discovery.

I thank news reporter Ake Spross of the *Upsala Nya Tidning* for locating and sharing with me his e-mail exchanges concerning the controversy associated with the awarding of the 2008 Nobel Prize. Steve Schulte, former director of the Los Angeles Gay and Lesbian Center, and Bill Misenhimer, former executive director of AIDS Project Los Angeles and first chief executive officer of amfAR, were extremely helpful in affording me the benefit of their insights concerning the inner workings of AIDS organizations. Don and Cindy Moran shared their insights into what transpired concerning AIDS within the Reagan White House. The current chief executive officer of amfAR, Kevin Robert Frost, took the time to explain to me his thinking in updating and correcting the organization's understanding of its history in preparation for its thirtieth anniversary in 2016. Jonathan Canno helped clarify actions taken by amfAR's board of directors.

Publishing a book is a team effort. My agent, Claire Gerus, applied her extensive knowledge and experience to guide me past some potentially poor choices of publishers to my relationship with ForeEdge, an imprint of the University Press of New England, and my excellent editor, Stephen Hull. Stephen taught me a great deal about how to keep readers on course and oriented to the story. I also thank my production editor, Peter Fong, for his encouragement and for his efforts to recover time lost in the production process.

Finally, I am grateful beyond words to three women who have had a profound effect on my writing. One is my twelfth-grade English teacher at Miami Beach Senior High School, Ann Hendricks, who first told me that she thought I had a talent for writing and encouraged me to develop it. A little encouragement can last a lifetime. Another is my second cousin, Merle Gordon, whose optimism in the face of serious difficulties I would hope to emulate. Merle's relating her experiences working in the dramatic arts in New York during the 1980s helped my understanding of the people and events of that era. Foremost, I am grateful to my wife, Pam Wexler, for her interest in and support of my writing. In particular, I am thankful for her patiently listening to me read to her each chapter of this book as it was written. The exercise may have put her to sleep at times, but her attention to detail and advice on what would be of greatest importance to readers was invaluable to my producing the best book of which I am capable.

NOTES

Introduction

1. Virologist Barbara Weiser's description of her first brush with the disease in late 1980 is an interesting example of how AIDS was viewed before Dr. Gottlieb described it as a new and distinct disease: "Henry Masur presented the first New York case [of AIDS] at intercity rounds. It was like 'stump the stars,' where people would present their mystery cases and everyone would try to guess what disease they had. . . . The last case [that evening in December 1980] was of a guard at Jacoby Hospital who had this lingering pneumonia which nobody could diagnose. . . . And finally the man had an open [lung] biopsy that showed *Pneumocystis*. At that time, the only people in the United States who had *Pneumocystis* [pneumonia] were people who were known to be immunosuppressed (i.e., their immune system was abnormal)."

2. A. M. Brandt, "Perspective: A Readers Guide to 200 Years of the *New England Journal of Medicine*," *New England Journal of Medicine* 366 (2012): 1–7.

ONE One Sick Queen

1. Author's interview with Dr. Michael Gottlieb, December 2014. Unless otherwise noted, all narrative, dialogue, and italicized thoughts attributed to Dr. Gottlieb in this chapter are derived from this interview.

2. Author's interview with Dr. Kenneth Shine, February 2015.

3. A herpetic whitlow is a painful infection of the fingertip caused by the herpes simplex virus.

4. An acute interstitial pneumonia, characterized by thick linear densities on a chest X-ray, is considered atypical and often attributable to an opportunistic infection.

5. Author's interview with Dr. Robert Wolf, April 2015. Unless otherwise noted, all narrative and dialogue attributed to Dr. Wolf in this chapter are based on this interview.

6. Dr. Gottlieb's recollection of what his patient said to a friend on the phone.

7. Identical antibodies with specific surface characteristics that facilitate their attachment to a specific biological target.

8. Oral history of Dr. Michael Gottlieb, Oral History Research Office, Columbia University, New York, 1999.

9. "Arnold Relman, Medicine's Long-Time Conscience, Dies at 91," *Medscape Medical News*, June 19, 2014, available at www.medscape.com/viewarticle/827038.

10. Dr. Gottlieb's recollection of what Dr. Elia said to him.

11. Dr. Gottlieb's recollection of his conversation with Dr. Arnold Relman.

12. M. Angell and J. P. Kassirer, "The Ingelfinger Rule Revisited," *New England Journal of Medicine* 325 (1991): 1371–1373.

13. Dr. Gottlieb's recollection of what Dr. Shandara said to him.

14. M. S. Gottlieb, H. M. Schanker, P. T. Fan, A. Saxon, and J. D. Weisman, "Pneumocystis Pneumonia—Los Angeles," *Morbidity and Mortality Weekly Report*, June 5, 1981, available at www.cdc.gov/mmwr/preview/mmwrhtml/june_5.htm.

15. "Kaposi's Sarcoma and Pneumocystis Pneumonia Among Homosexual Men—New York City and California," *Morbidity and Mortality Weekly Report*, July 3, 1981 (abstract available at www.popline.org/node/419814).

16. L. K. Altman, "Rare Cancer Seen in 41 Homosexuals," *New York Times*, July 3, 1981, available at www.nytimes.com/1981/07/03/us/rare-cancer-seen-in-41-homosexuals.html.

17. Interview with Cindy (Gottlieb) Sapp, December 2014. All dialogue in this chapter attributed to Ms. Sapp is derived from this interview.

18. M. S. Gottlieb, R. Schroff, H. M. Schanker, et al., "*Pneumosystis Carinii* Pneumonia and Mucosal *Candidiasis* in Previously Healthy Homosexual Men—Evidence of a New Acquired Cellular Immunodeficiency," *New England Journal of Medicine* 305 (1981): 1425–1431.

19. John Fahey's online memoir, available at www.johnfaheymd.com/?page_id=549.

20. A timeline of the development of HIV/AIDS is available at en.wikipedia.org/wiki/Timeline_of_HIV/AIDS.

21. M. S. Gottlieb, "Discovering AIDS," *Epidemiology* 9 (1998): 365–367.

TWO Riding the Tiger

1. Author's interview with Dr. Michael Gottlieb, December 2014. Unless otherwise noted, all narrative, dialogue, and italicized thoughts attributed to Dr. Gottlieb in this chapter are derived from this interview.

2. Author's interview with Dr. Andrew Saxon, March 2015. Unless otherwise noted, all dialogue attributed to Dr. Saxon in this chapter is derived from this interview.

3. M. S. Gottlieb, R. Schroff, and H. M. Schanker, "Pneumosystis Carinii Pneumonia and Mucosal Candidiasis in Previously Healthy Homosexual Men—

Evidence of a New Acquired Cellular Immunodeficiency," *New England Journal of Medicine* 305 (1981): 1425–1431.

4. Dr. Saxon may have erred in this regard, as the only patients referred from outside the hospital among the series of patients Gottlieb reported on in his *NEJM* article came from Joel Weisman, with whom he met in person prior to the patients' transfer to UCLA.

5. A granuloma is an advanced, consolidated focus of infection.

6. What Dr. Saxon may have been recalling was, according to Dr. Gottlieb, whitlow, a manifestation of herpes infection, which was present on both index fingers.

7. Author's interview with Dr. Robert Wolf, April 2015. All narrative and dialogue attributed to Dr. Wolf in this chapter are derived from this interview.

8. Author's interview with Dr. Kenneth Shine, March 2015. All narrative and dialogue attributed to Dr. Shine in this chapter are derived from this interview.

9. Author's interview with Dr. Martin Shapiro, March 2015.

10. "Art Gottlieb," *Jews in Sports*, n.d., available at www.jewsinsports.org/profile .asp?sport=football&ID=198.

11. Oral history of Dr. Michael Gottlieb, Oral History Research Office, Columbia University, New York, 1999.

12. Oral history of Dr. Michael Gottlieb.

13. Author's interview with Dr. John Hanks, December 2014.

14. Author's interview with Ms. Cynthia (Gottlieb) Sapp, December 2014. Unless otherwise noted, all narrative and dialogue attributed to Ms. Sapp in this chapter are derived from this interview.

15. Dr. Gottlieb's recollection of what Dr. James DeWeese said to him.

16. Feedback loops are bodily mechanisms for sensing how much of a substance, like a hormone or protein, the body is producing and informing the responsible organ to make more or less of it.

17. Dr. Gottlieb's recollection of what Dr. John Condemi said to him.

18. Photocopy of a letter from Drs. Kenneth Shine and Andrew Saxon to Dean A. Frederick Rasmussen Jr., May 5, 1980 (from Dr. Gottlieb's UCLA employment file).

19. Dr. Gottlieb's recollection of what Dr. Kenneth Shine said to him.

20. Dr. Michael Gottlieb, personal communication, January 2016.

21. R. Shilts, *And the Band Played On* (New York: St. Martin's Press, 1987).

THREE Fast Times

1. To protect the identity of actual patients who provided their stories and gave permission to use their input into the narrative and their verbatim dialogue, Brad

Hartley is an amalgam of individuals interviewed by the author from December 2014 through August 2015.

2. Prior to recognition that the syndrome could affect heterosexual men and women and to its being renamed AIDS, the disease was referred to as GRID, for "gay-related immune deficiency."

3. Quoted in "Continental Baths," *Wikipedia*, n.d., available at en.wikipedia.org /wiki/Continental_Baths.

4. Chris Geidner, "13 Times the White House Press Briefing Erupted with Laughter Over AIDS," *BuzzFeed News*, December 2, 2013, available at www.buzzfeed .com/chrisgeidner/times-the-reagan-white-house-press-briefing-erupted -with#.ae6ZRGJJE.

5. "Timeline of HIV/AIDS," *Wikipedia*, n.d., available at https//:en.wikipedia .org/wiki/Timeline_of_HIV/AIDS.

6. "The Historic Stonewall Inn," n.d., available at www.thestonewallinnnyc. com/StonewallInnNYC/HISTORY.html; "Introduction: Stonewall Uprising," *The American Experience*, available at www.pbs.org/wgbh/americanexperience /features/introduction/stonewall-intro/.

7. "Jerry Falwell," *Wikiquote*, n.d., available at en.wikiquote.org/wiki/Jerry _Falwell.

8. "Jerry Falwell."

9. Author's e-mail exchange with Donald W. Moran, who served in several positions in the Reagan White House during 1981–1985, October 2015.

FOUR The Waxman Cometh

1. T. Westmoreland, "Henry Waxman, the Unsung Hero in the Fight Against AIDS," *Politico*, February 4, 2014, available at www.politico.com/magazine /story/2014/02/henry-waxman-aids-fight-103123.html#.VO-bNdhoy7o.

2. J. Green, "The Heroic Story of How Congress First Confronted AIDS," *The Atlantic*, June 8, 2011, available at www.theatlantic.com/politics/archive/2011/06 /the-heroic-story-of-how-congress-first-confronted-aids/240131/.

3. "William E. Dannemeyer," *Wikipedia*, n.d., available at en.wikipedia.org /wiki/William_E._Dannemeyer.

4. J. E. Groopman and M. S. Gottlieb, "Kaposi's Sarcoma: An Oncologic Looking Glass," *Nature* 299 (1982): 103–104.

5. Westmoreland, "Henry Waxman, the Unsung Hero in the Fight Against AIDS."

6. R. Shilts, *And the Band Played On* (New York: Saint Martin's Press, 1987).

7. Photocopy of a letter from Dr. Andrew Saxon and Department of Medicine

vice chair Dr. Robert Sparkes to Dean A. Frederick Rasmussen Jr., January 29, 1982 (from Dr. Gottlieb's UCLA employment file).

8. Author's interview with Dr. Andrew Saxon, March 2015. Unless otherwise noted, all dialogue attributed to Dr. Saxon in this chapter is derived from this interview.

9. Author's interview with Dr. Peter Wolfe, March 2015. Unless otherwise noted, all narrative and dialogue attributed to Dr. Wolf in this chapter are derived from this interview.

10. Author's interview with Ms. Cynthia (Gottlieb) Sapp, December 2014. Unless otherwise noted, all dialogue attributed to Ms. Sapp in this chapter is derived from this interview.

11. J. E. Groopman and M. S. Gottlieb, "AIDS: The Widening Gyre," *Nature* 303 (1983): 575-576.

12. Author's interview with Dr. Samuel Broder. Unless otherwise noted, all narrative and dialogue attributed to Dr. Broder in this chapter are derived from this interview.

13. Jon Cohen AIDS Research Collection, n.d., available at quod.lib.umich. edu/c/cohenaids/browse.html.

FIVE The Color of Money

1. Dr. Gottlieb's recollection of what Dr. Marcus Conant said to him on the phone. Author's interview with Dr. Michael Gottlieb, February 2015.

2. "Willie Brown Biography," n.d., available at www.biography.com/people /willie-brown-40059; "Willie Brown (politician)," *Wikipedia*, n.d., available at. en.wikipedia.org/wiki/Willie_Brown_(politician).

3. Author's interview with Dr. Michael Gottlieb, February 2014. Unless otherwise noted, all narrative, dialogue, and italicized thoughts attributed to Dr. Gottlieb in this chapter are derived from this interview.

4. Photocopy of a letter from Dr. Gottlieb to Dr. Shine, April 28, 1983 (from Dr. Gottlieb).

5. Photocopy of a letter from Dr. Shine to Dr. Gottlieb, May 5, 1983 (from Dr. Gottlieb).

6. Indirect costs are dollars paid over and above the requested budget to do the actual research. "Indirect cost reimbursement," as it is called, pays the institution for the expense of space, heat, administrative personnel, IT, and numerous other services necessary to conduct the research.

7. Dr. Gottlieb's recollection of what Dr. Conant told him about a phone call he had received from Dr. Golde, confirmed by Dr. Conant in an e-mail, October 31, 2015.

8. Photocopy of a letter from the university system administrative offices to Dr. Gottlieb, received June 3, 1983 (from Dr. Gottlieb).

9. Dr. Gottlieb's recollection of what Dr. Shine said to him on the specific occasion described.

10. Photocopy of a letter from Dr. Golde to Dr. Sande, June 21, 1984 (from Dr. Gottlieb).

11. Photocopy of a letter from Dr. Golde to Dr. Gottlieb, June 25, 1984 (from Dr. Gottlieb).

12. Oral history of Dr. Michael Gottlieb, Oral History Research Office, Columbia University, New York, 1999.

13. The events surrounding the discovery of HTLV-III and its similarity to the virus LAV (later renamed HIV), discovered by a French team some months earlier, would eventually embroil Gottlieb in the race between American and French laboratories to identify the cause of AIDS.

14. Author's interview with Ms. Kathryn Petersilie, February 2015. Unless otherwise noted, all dialogue attributed to Ms. Petersilie in this chapter is taken verbatim from this interview.

15. Oral history of Dr. Michael Gottlieb.

16. Roger Horowitz's dying from AIDS was the subject of Paul Monette's *Borrowed Time*.

17. Dr. Gottlieb's recollection of what Dr. Shine said to him on the specific occasion described.

18. Oral history of Dr. Michael Gottlieb.

SIX No Love Lost

1. W. C. Greene, "A History of AIDS: Looking Back to See Ahead," *European Journal of Immunology* 37 (November 2007): S94–S102, available at onlinelibrary.wiley.com/doi/10.1002/eji.200737441/full.

2. Author's interview with Drs. Barbara Weiser and Harold Burger in March 2015. Unless otherwise noted, all dialogue attributed to Drs. Weiser and Burger in this chapter is taken verbatim from this interview.

3. HTLV-I was the first human retrovirus ever isolated. It was discovered by Dr. Robert Gallo and his laboratory at the NIH. The virus was already known to be the cause of a rare type of leukemia and of a Caribbean neurologic disease, tropical spastic paraparesis.

4. Recollection of Dr. Barbara Weiser of what Dr. John-Claude Chermont said to her in 1984 (from interview with Drs. Weiser and Burger).

5. J. Crewdson, "The Great AIDS Quest: Science Under the Microscope," *Chicago*

Tribune, November 19, 1989, available at archives.chicagotribune.com/1989/11/19/page/101/article/the-great-aids-quest.

6. Despite the threat, Gardner participated in the French investigation in Africa.

7. J. Levy, "Isolation of Lymphocytopathic Retroviruses from San Francisco Patients with AIDS," *Science* 225 (1984): 840-842.

8. P. Strudwick, "I Look Like a Virus, My Face Is Like HIV: A Conversation with Françoise Barré-Sinoussi," *Pacific Standard*, June 16, 2014, available at www.psmag.com/health-and-behavior/hiv-aids-discovery-disease-conversation-francoise-barre-sinoussi-83571.

9. Strudwick, "I Look Like a Virus."

10. Crewdson, "The Great AIDS Quest."

11. A. Vahlne, "A Historical Reflection on the Discovery of Human Retroviruses," *Retrovirology* 6 (2009): 40-49.

12. All materials concerning the deliberations leading to the awarding of a Nobel Prize, including the names of nominees, are sequestered for fifty years.

13. M. L. Lever and B. Berkhout, "Nobel Prize in Medicine for Discoverers of HIV," *Retrovirology* 5 (2008): 91-92.

14. Author's interview with Dr. Andrew Saxon, March 2015.

15. "Ceremonies Archive, 2008," Nobelprize.org, 2016, available at www.nobelprize.org/ceremonies/archive/.

16. The Nobel Prize in Physiology or Medicine 2008, available at http://www.nobelprize.org/nobel_prizes/medicine/laureates/2008/.

17. "Nobel Banquet Menu 2008," Nobelprize.org, 2016, available at www.nobelprize.org/ceremonies/menus/menu-2008.html.

18. Françoise Barré-Sinoussi, "HIV: A Discovery Opening the Road to Novel Scientific Knowledge and Global Health Improvement" (presented at the Karolinska Institute, Stockholm Sweden, December 7, 2008), available at www.nobelprize.org/nobel_prizes/medicine/laureates/2008/barre-sinoussi-lecture.html.

19. E-mails between Ake Spross and Michael Gottlieb, 2008 (from Mr. Spross).

20. Strudwick, "I Look Like a Virus."

21. Strudwick, "I Look Like a Virus."

SEVEN The Power of Denial

1. A mixture of cocaine and heroin, popular among some gay men.

2. C. Kalinga, "The Responsibility of Memorializing Sex, the Dying and the Dead in HIV/AIDS Drama: Larry Kramer's *The Normal Heart* and William Hoffman's *As Is*," *STET: An Online Postgraduate Research Journal* 4 (May 2014): 1-26.

3. Author's interview with Dr. Marcus A. Conant, April 2015. All references to Dr. Conant's thoughts and actions in this chapter are derived from this interview.

EIGHT Rock

1. Author's interview with Dr. Michael Gottlieb, April 2015. Unless otherwise noted, all narrative and dialogue attributed to Dr. Gottlieb in this chapter are derived from this interview.

2. Author's interview with Ms. Kathryn Petersilie, February 2015. Unless otherwise noted, all dialogue attributed to Ms. Petersilie in this chapter is taken verbatim from this interview.

3. E. McNeil, "Rock Hudson's 'True Love' Speaks: How We Kept Our Gay Love Secret," *People*, April 15, 2015, available at http://www.people.com/article/rock-hudson-boyfriend-lee-garlington-gay-life.

4. "Rock Hudson," *Wikipedia*, n.d., available at en.wikipedia.org/wiki/Rock_Hudson.

5. E. McNeil, "The Untold Story: Rock's Final Days," *People*, April 27, 2015, 70–74.

6. "Rock Hudson."

7. McNeil, "The Untold Story."

8. McNeil, "The Untold Story."

9. Dr. Michael Gottlieb's recollection of what Pierre Salinger said to him on the phone (from interview with Dr. Gottlieb, April 2015).

10. Author's interview with Dr. Kenneth Shine, March 2015. All dialogue and narrative attributed to Dr. Shine in this chapter is derived from that interview.

11. "Rock Hudson."

12. Soon after Hudson's death, Gottlieb made a video with Morgan Fairchild promoting safe sex. The video drew considerable attention and a death threat, as well as numerous letters touting home remedies for HIV/AIDS.

13. "Rock Hudson."

14. News Services, "Friend Says Hudson Was Unaware of His Role in Fight against AIDS," *San Diego Union*, October 5, 1985.

15. P. C. B. Allens, "Colleagues Stand, Saddened on Learning of Hudson's Death," *Evening Outlook*, October 3, 1985.

16. Allens, "Colleagues Stand."

17. Allens, "Colleagues Stand."

18. R. Shilts, *And the Band Played On* (New York: Saint Martin's Press, 1987).

19. "Timeline of HIV/AIDS," *Wikipedia*, n.d., available at https//:en.wikipedia.org/wiki/Timeline_of_HIV/AIDS. In 1988 Koop was responsible for the

government sending a condensed version of his full report, titled *Understanding AIDS*, to every household in the United States.

20. Shilts, *And the Band Played On*.

21. N. Collins, "Liz's AIDS Odyssey," *Vanity Fair*, October 31, 1992, available at www.vanityfair.com/news/1992/11/elizabeth-taylor-activism-aids.

22. A. White, "Reagan's AIDS Legacy/Silence Equals Death," *SF Gate*, June 8, 2004, available at www.sfgate.com/opinion/openforum/article/Reagan-s-AIDS-Legacy-Silence-equals-death-2751030.php.

23. NIH frequently calls for grant applications on a specific topic by setting aside monies and announcing an RFA. Such was the case with this particular AIDS research opportunity.

24. Photocopy of letter from Dr. Michael Gottlieb to Dr. John Fahey, August 20, 1985 (from Dr. Gottlieb).

25. Dr. Kenneth Shine's recollection of what Dr. Gottlieb said during the conversation.

26. The expression is a common one in the film community, meaning ingratiating one's self with celebrities in the hopes that some of the glamour will rub off on one.

NINE Elizabeth

1. Author's interview with Dr. Andrew Saxon, March 2015. Unless otherwise noted, all narrative and dialogue attributed to Dr. Saxon in this chapter are derived from this interview.

2. Author's interview with Dr. Michael Gottlieb, April 2015.

3. Taylor converted to Judaism in 1957, coincident with her marriage to Michael Todd.

4. Quoted in "Elizabeth Taylor," *Wikipedia*, n.d., available at en.wikipedia.org/wiki/Elizabeth_Taylor.

5. "Who's Afraid of Virginia Woolf," *Wikipedia*, n.d., available at en.wikipedia.org/wiki/Who%27s_Afraid_of_Virginia_Woolf%3F_(film).

6. E. McNeil, "The Untold Story: Rock's Final Days," *People*, April 27, 2015, 70–74.

7. N. Collins, "Liz's AIDS Odyssey," *Vanity Fair*, October 31, 1992, available at www.vanityfair.com/news/1992/11/elizabeth-taylor-activism-aids.

8. Collins, "Liz's AIDS Odyssey."

9. Author's interview with Bill Misenhimer, May 2015. Unless otherwise noted, all narrative and dialogue attributed to Mr. Misenhimer in this chapter are derived from this interview.

10. Collins, "Liz's AIDS Odyssey."

11. Collins, "Liz's AIDS Odyssey."

12. The Elizabeth Taylor AIDS Foundation, "Timeline," 2015, available at elizabethtayloraidsfoundation.org/timeline/#.

13. The benefit originally was supposed to take place in Century City, but overwhelming demand required the organizers to move the event to the downtown Bonaventure Hotel. Even so, people had to be turned away for lack of space.

14. In 1991 Roger Wall committed suicide after learning that he had contracted AIDS. Ms. Taylor said that her assistant's death was one of the greatest losses of her life.

15. Collins, "Liz's AIDS Odyssey."

16. Collins, "Liz's AIDS Odyssey."

17. Collins, "Liz's AIDS Odyssey."

18. Ruth Schwartz Cowan, "Mathilde Krim," Jewish Women's Archive Encyclopedia, n.d., available at jwa.org/encyclopedia/article/krim-matilde.

19. "Mathilde Krim," *Wikipedia*, n.d., available at en.wikipedia.org/wiki/Mathilde_Krim.

20. Both Beirn and Decker later died of AIDS.

21. Mathilde Krim declined to be interviewed, citing poor health.

22. Author's interview with Jonathan Canno, September 2015.

23. Collins, "Liz's AIDS Odyssey."

24. P. C. B. Allens, "Foundation to Raise AIDS Funds," *Torrance Daily Breeze*, September 27, 1985.

25. Collins, "Liz's AIDS Odyssey."

26. Photocopies of memos from Dr. Andrew Saxon to Dr. Michael Gottlieb, July 17, 1986, and August 1, 1986 (from Dr. Gottlieb).

27. For academic physicians, matters are a little more complex. What is guaranteed is a portion of the physician's salary; however, the amount is most often quite small. A reduction in salary to the guaranteed level usually encourages the physician to leave the institution.

28. January 1984 report of the Council on Academic Personnel on the performance of Dr. Michael Gottlieb (from Dr. Gottlieb's UCLA employment file).

29. Photocopy of a letter from Associate Dean John G. Pierce, PhD, to Dr. Kenneth Shine, June 14, 1984 (from Dr. Gottlieb's UCLA employment file).

30. Photocopy of a letter from Drs. Andrew Saxon and Kenneth Shine to Associate Dean Irving Zabin, MD, December 12, 1985 (from Dr. Gottlieb's UCLA employment file).

31. The origins of this expression are uncertain.

TEN The Contentious Route to an Effective Treatment

1. The first antibody test kits for AIDS were approved in March 1985. They were immediately applied to testing for HIV in community blood supplies. "Timeline of HIV/AIDS." *Wikipedia*, n.d. available at https//:en.wikipedia.org/wiki/Timeline _of_HIV/AIDS.

2. Photocopy of a letter from Dr. Frank Apgar to Dr. Michael Gottlieb, July 7, 1986 (from Dr. Gottlieb).

3. Letter from Dr. Michael Gottlieb to Dr. Frank Apgar, July 28, 1986 (from Dr. Gottlieb).

4. S. Broder, "The Development of Antiretroviral Therapy and Its Impact on the HIV-1/AIDS Pandemic," *Antiviral Research* 85 (2010): 1–18.

5. Oral history of Dr. Michael Gottlieb, Oral History Research Office, Columbia University, New York, 1999.

6. African trypanisomiasis is a parasitic disease. Transmission of the parasite to humans occurs via the bite of the tsetse fly.

7. Pharmaceutical companies often point to the amount of time over which they are investing money in the research and assessment of a new drug, as opposed to investing the money elsewhere, as the most significant cost of drug development. This is known as the opportunity cost.

8. The author worked part-time as the chief science officer of an imaging CRO, ACR Image Metrix, during the period 2007–2013.

9. Joel Weisman, DO, had been an author on Gottlieb's original article on AIDS in *NEJM*.

10. Broder, "Development of Antiretroviral Therapy."

11. Trials aimed at proving efficacy usually have "stopping rules" as part of the trial design to ensure that if the trial shows a decidedly negative result while the study is ongoing, subjects can be protected from having to take unnecessary or even harmful medications. Conversely, with early stopping for a positive result, patients assigned to the control arm can begin taking the effective drug.

12. Large randomized clinical trials usually have a data safety monitoring board to ensure that the trial is conducted ethically and adverse events are properly noted, and to review data as they are accumulated. Members of a DSMB are the only ones allowed to see the data during the trial and may not have any other role in the trial. One of the DSMB functions is to stop the trial if either a positive or negative outcome becomes obvious earlier than expected.

13. S. Broder, "The Development of Antiretroviral Therapy and Its Impact on the HIV-1/AIDS Pandemic," *Antiviral Research* 85 (2010): 1–18.

14. Broder, "Development of Antiretroviral Therapy."

ELEVEN Fear Itself

1. FDA approval to market the first test kits was granted in March 1985.

2. David L. Kirp, "LaRouche Turns to AIDS Politics," *New York Times*, September 11, 1986.

3. LaRouche never managed to persuade even 1 percent of the electorate to vote for him.

4. "Lyndon LaRouche," *Wikipedia*, n.d., available at en.wikipedia.org/wiki /Lyndon_LaRouche#1985.E2.80.931986:_PANIC.2C_LaRouche.27s_AIDS _initiative.

5. Author's interview with Dr. Michael Gottlieb, June 2015.

6. Author's interview with Dr. Andrew Saxon, March 2015.

7. Author's interview with Bill Misenhimer, May 2015.

8. Hemophilia encompasses genetic disorders wherein the body fails to produce one or another "factor" needed for normal blood clotting, so that even minor injuries can put an affected individual at risk of excessive blood loss. The treatment involves providing the missing factor derived from blood products.

9. *Hearings before the House Subcommittee on Health and the Environment of the Committee on Energy and Commerce*, 99th Cong., July 22, 1985, 58–59.

10. Photocopy of a letter from UCLA Administrator Brad H. Volkmer to Michael Gottlieb, MD, July 5, 1984 (from Dr. Gottlieb).

11. Author's interview with Ms. Cynthia (Gottlieb) Sapp, December 2014.

12. Photocopy of a memo from Dr. David Golde to a number of UCLA faculty, February 21, 1986 (from Dr. Gottlieb).

13. Photocopy of a letter from Dr. Kenneth Shine to Dr. Gottlieb, March 31, 1986 (from Dr. Gottlieb).

14. Photocopy of a letter from Drs. Michael Gottlieb, Ronald Mitsuyasu, Andrew Saxon, and Peter Wolf to Cornelius L. Hopper, October 29, 1985 (from Dr. Gottlieb).

15. Photocopy of a letter from Dr. Michael Gottlieb to Dr. David Golde, March 27, 1986 (from Dr. Gottlieb).

16. Photocopy of a letter from Dr. Kenneth Shine to Dr. Michael Gottlieb, March 31, 1986 (from Dr. Gottlieb).

17. Photocopy of a letter from Dr. Michael Gottlieb to Dr. David Golde, April 24, 1986 (from Dr. Gottlieb).

18. Photocopy of a letter from Dr. Michael Gottlieb to Brad Volkmer, April 24, 1986 (from Dr. Gottlieb).

19. Photocopy of a letter from Dr. Michael Gottlieb to Dr. David Golde, August 5, 1986 (from Dr. Gottlieb).

20. Photocopy of a letter from Dr. Michael Gottlieb to Dr. Esther Hays, chair of the Dean's Advisory Committee on AIDS, October 23, 1986 (from Dr. Gottlieb).

TWELVE The Politics of Research Advocacy

1. Oral history of Dr. Michael Gottlieb, Oral History Research Office, Columbia University, New York, 1999.

2. Photocopy of Ms. Taylor's 1986 address to Congress (from Dr. Gottlieb).

3. Author's interview with Dr. Michael Gottlieb, May 2015. Unless otherwise noted, all narrative and dialogue attributed to Dr. Gottlieb in this chapter is derived from this interview.

4. Given the national media frenzy surrounding Elizabeth Taylor's press conference, with both Gottlieb and Krim at her side, it is hard to imagine that Dr. Shine had not previously heard anything about Gottlieb's involvement in amfAR. He may have meant that this was the first occasion on which he had discussed it with Dr. Gottlieb.

5. There was no such position in amfAR. Dr. Shine probably was referring to Gottlieb's chairing amfAR's Scientific Advisory Committee.

6. Author's interview with Dr. Kenneth Shine, March 2015. Unless otherwise noted, all narrative and dialogue attributed to Dr. Shine in this chapter are derived from this interview.

7. It wasn't until 1991, after the basketball player Magic Johnson announced he was HIV-infected, that UCLA developed a home for AIDS in the institution.

8. Author's interview with Bill Misenhimer, May 2015.

9. E-mail from Dr. Gottlieb to the author, November 8, 2015.

10. Photocopy of a memo from Dr. Michael Gottlieb to Dr. Mathilde Krim, May 12, 1986 (from Dr. Gottlieb).

11. Photocopy of a letter from Dr. Michael Gottlieb to Dr. Mathilde Krim, December 24, 1986 (from Dr. Gottlieb).

12. V. J. Barker, "AIDS Researcher Offers Idea on How Disease Got to U.S.," *Ogden Standard-Examiner*, October 26, 1988.

13. The author founded one of these groups, the American College of Radiology Imaging Network (ACRIN), and led it for nine years.

14. Oral history of Dr. Michael Gottlieb.

15. "Mathilde Krim," *Wikipedia*, n.d., available at https://en.wikipedia.org/wiki/Mathilde_Krim.

THIRTEEN The Making of a Radical

1. "ACT UP," *Wikipedia*, n.d., available at https://en.wikipedia.org/wiki/ACT_UP.

2. Larry Kramer interview, November 15, 2003, in *ACT UP Oral History Project* (The New York Lesbian & Gay Experimental Film Festival, Inc., 2004), available at www.actuporalhistory.org/interviews/images/kramer.pdf.

3. Larry Kramer interview.

4. A. M. Petro, "After the Wrath of God: AIDS, Sexuality, and American Religion" (PhD thesis, Princeton University, 2011).

5. Larry Kramer interview.

FOURTEEN *Le Deluge*

1. Author's interview with Dr. Michael Gottlieb, June 2015. Unless otherwise noted, all dialogue and narrative attributed to Dr. Gottlieb in this chapter are derived from this interview.

2. Oral history of Dr. Michael Gottlieb, Oral History Research Office, Columbia University, New York, 1999.

3. Photocopy of a letter from Dr. Michael Gottlieb to Dr. Andrew Saxon, March 31, 1986 (from Dr. Gottlieb).

4. Photocopy of a letter from Dr. Michael Gottlieb to Dr. Andrew Saxon, April 23, 1986 (from Dr. Gottlieb).

5. Photocopy of a letter from Dr. Michael Gottlieb to Dr. Maureen Myers at NIAID, October 14, 1986 (from Dr. Gottlieb).

6. Undated memo from Dr. Michael Gottlieb to Dr. Andrew Saxon.

7. Photocopy of a letter from Dr. Michael Gottlieb to Dr. Andrew Saxon, October 25, 1986 (from Dr. Gottlieb).

8. Photocopy of a letter from Dr. Andrew Saxon to Dr. Michael Gottlieb, October 27, 1986 (from Dr. Gottlieb).

9. Dr. Shine was referring to his having to intervene when Gottlieb initially had not included Wolf as an author on his *NEJM* manuscript in 1981.

10. Author's interview with Dr. Kenneth Shine, March 2015. All narrative and dialogue attributed to Dr. Shine in this chapter are derived from this interview.

11. Gottlieb did not recall Dr. Shine ever mentioning to him that a problem existed in his dealings with colleagues over authorship of AIDS-related publications. In rebuttal, he offered examples of several instances in which he might have had a reasonable case to claim authorship but had not done so.

12. Dr. Shine was referring to the NIAID request for proposals that eventually was awarded to UCLA.

13. Author's interview with Ms. Cynthia (Gottlieb) Sapp, December 2014. Unless otherwise noted, all narrative and dialogue attributed to Ms. Sapp in this chapter are derived from this interview.

14. The author is a 1985 graduate of the RAND/UCLA program. Although he and Dr. Gottlieb were both in Los Angeles during 1985, they had no contact.

15. Dr. Gottlieb's recollection of his conversation with Dr. Williams.

16. Oral history of Dr. Michael Gottlieb, Oral History Research Office, Columbia University, New York, 1999.

17. Oral history of Dr. Michael Gottlieb.

18. Oral history of Dr. Michael Gottlieb.

19. Photocopy of a letter from Dr. Michael Gottlieb to the chairman of the board of AIDS Project Los Angeles, July 7, 1986 (from Dr. Gottlieb).

20. Photocopy of a letter and list of names and addresses from Dr. Michael Gottlieb to Dr. Andrew Saxon, August 11, 1986 (from Dr. Gottlieb).

21. Author's interview with Dr. Martin Shapiro, during March 2015.

22. A. M. Brandt, "A Reader's Guide to 200 Years of the *New England Journal of Medicine*," *New England Journal of Medicine* 366 (2012): 1–5.

23. Author's interview with Dr. Peter Wolfe, March 2015.

24. Photocopy of Dr. Gottlieb's letter of resignation from the full-time UCLA faculty, March 16, 1987 (from Dr. Gottlieb).

25. H. Nelson, "Dr. Who Reported 1st AIDS Victims Resigns UCLA Post," *Los Angeles Times*, April 30, 1987.

26. Oral history of Dr. Michael Gottlieb.

27. Oral history of Dr. Michael Gottlieb.

EPILOGUE

1. Author's interview with Jillian Gottlieb, August 2015.

2. Author's interview with Dr. Michael Gottlieb and subsequent e-mail exchanges, July–August 2015. Unless otherwise noted, all narrative and dialogue attributed to Dr. Gottlieb in this chapter are derived from these communications.

3. Author's interview with an AIDS patient cared for by Dr. Michael Gottlieb, January 2015. Unless otherwise noted, all narrative and dialogue attributed to the patient in this chapter are derived from this interview.

4. For detailed information about the development of AIDS therapies and a time line, see S. Broder, "The Development of Anti-retroviral Therapy and Its Impact on the HIV-1/AIDS Pandemic," *Antiviral Research* 85 (2010): 1–18; "Timeline of HIV/AIDS," Wikipedia, n.d., available at https://en.wikipedia.org/wiki/Timeline_of _HIV/AIDS.

5. "Overview of HIV Treatments," available at https://www.aids.gov/hiv-aids -basics/just-diagnosed-hiv-aids/treatment-options.

6. The American Foundation for AIDS Research shortened its name to the Foundation for AIDS Research in 2005 but retained the acronym amfAR. amfAR: Making Aids History, "Introduction and History," n.d., available at http://www .amfar.org/About-amfAR/Introduction-and-History/.

7. M. Shapiro, "Residents' Experiences in, and Attitudes Toward, the Care of Persons with AIDS in Canada, France, and the United States." *Journal of the American Medical Association* 268 (1992): 510–518.

8. "The History of the HIV/AIDS Virus," n.d., available at www.healthline.com /health/hiv-aids/history-of-the-aids-virus.

9. World Health Organization, Global Health Observatory (GHO) Data: HIV. AIDS, n.d., available at www.who.int/gho/hiv/en.

10. "The History of the HIV/AIDS Virus," n.d., available at www.healthline.com /health/hiv-aids/history-of-the-aids-virus.